MW00781237

Grandma Bell's

A to Z Guide to

HEALING

with

HERBS

Grandma Bell's
A to Z Guide to
HEALING
with
HERBS

Copyright © 1995, 2003
by
William Campbell Douglass, MD

All rights reserved. Copyright under Berne Copyright Convention, Universal Copyright Convention, and Pan-American Copyright Convention. No part of this book may be reproduced, stored in a retrieval system, or transmitted in any form, or by any means, electronic, mechanical, photocopying, recording or otherwise, without prior written permission of the publisher and author.

ISBN 9962-636-12-4

Cover illustration by
Alex Manyoma (alex@3dcity.com)

Please, visit Rhino's website for other publications from
Dr. William Campbell Douglass
www.rhinopublish.com

Dr. Douglass' "Real Health" alternative medical
newsletter is available at www.realhealthnews.com

RHINO PUBLISHING, S.A.
World Trade Center
Panama, Republic of Panama
Voicemail/Fax
International: + 416-352-5126
North America: 888-317-6767

Dedication

To Lucy McDaniel Bell, physician and healer

Acknowledgments

Writing a book about my great-grandmother has been an extremely rewarding endeavor and I owe a great deal of gratitude to the woman who made it possible, Lucy McDaniel Bell. Obviously, without her this book would never have been written.

But there were several other people who made this book what it is today. First, I'd like to say "thank you" to my Uncle John. The time he spent through the years telling me stories about Grandma Bell have enriched my life and added a new dimension to my medical career.

Next is my publisher and good friend, Chip Wood, who first encouraged me to write this book and kept prodding me until it was done.

I also wish to thank my former tennis partner and patient research assistant, Nick Lester, for his many hours of advice and assistance.

And finally, but certainly not least, I wish to express a special word of appreciation to my editor, Steve Kroening, who never revolted during the many cuts, edits, and rewrites, and worked tirelessly to see this project through to completion. His vision, expertise, and hard work helped make Grandma Bell come to life again in these pages.

For the assistance, encouragement, and inspiraton of all of you, I am truly grateful.

Table of Contents

Introduction

The Local War Hero

Lucy McDaniel Bell was my great grand-mother. She lived in the Georgia mountains, 50 miles north of Atlanta, in a village called Ball Ground. This town of a few hundred mountaineers was named after an old Cherokee Indian playing field where the forerunner of American baseball was played. Lucy was an herbalist and the only doctor in those parts— 50 miles of dirt roads made Atlanta a long horse-and-buggy ride away.

Her face was thin and the eyes were a glistening black, especially when she was amused, which was often, although I never heard her actually laugh. She always wore a print skirt down to her black shoes and her hair was pinned back in a careless bun, as a sort of an afterthought.

I don't know how much schooling she got, probably not much. She learned herbal medicine from the remaining Cherokee Indians, or from people who had known the Indians, mostly the latter. By the time the War Between the States started in 1861, Lucy was a child and almost all the Indians had been pushed West.

Lucy became a local hero at the age of eight. When General W. T. Sherman came through Ball Ground on his way to burning Atlanta, he rode up to the small hotel, dismounted, and asked the little girl on the boardwalk to take his horse. It was scrawny little Lucy he had asked, and she refused, saying she wouldn't hold the horse of a damn Yankee invader. Lucy's black nanny quickly took the reins of the horse and apologized to the general. He laughed with gusto and entered the hotel.

I don't know if the story is true or not, but I do know the legend of Lucy Bell began with tales of this encounter between the conqueror of the South and a little eight-year-old girl. Sherman was said to have been very amused by the incident. Lucy didn't think it was funny and, to the day she died, she "would have no truck with

Yankees." When Sherman left, contrary to his custom, he ordered the hotel to be spared the torch.

When fully grown Lucy weighed about 90 pounds in her goulashes, with her winter coat on. She lived to be 99 and if there ever was an incarnation of Mammy Yokum, Lucy was it.

This book is my tribute to my wise great-grandmother, affectionately known to the Douglass clan as Grandma Bell. Oh, if I had only listened to her when she was around. But like most young know-it-alls, I thought I was the font of modern scientific wisdom.

Foolish boy that I was, my faith was firmly planted in the church of science. Of course, when you worship at those feet you are not only worshiping double-blind studies, scientific reasoning, and the glory of the AMA, but you're kneeling at the altar of the new. Everything new is scientific — it's good. Everything old is pre-science, outdated science, or — worst of all — old wives' tales, and *bad.*

So for years I thought Grandma Bell's wonderful mixture of Americana medicine and old-world cures were silly and stupid — more of the age of Mark Twain than the age of Truman and Eisenhower. I would listen and promptly forget most of what she had to say. After all, I was a doctor, a young new doctor fresh from medical school and cock-sure of my knowledge and abilities.

Grandma Bell, forgive me. You were right; I was wrong. All it took for me to see your wisdom was the needless death of patients who were killed by scientifically proven drugs and scientifically accepted techniques. I watched my colleagues ignore common-sense evidence and make the most absurd diagnoses, simply because they insisted on following scientific procedures and ignoring common sense.

I did the same, until the weight of evidence and the weight on my heart forced me to look, for the first time, at the wisdom of traditional home remedies and the value of my own good old American common-sense.

What a revelation! Once you wake up from the stupor of scientific theology and clear your head of the constant propaganda spewing forth from greedy drug companies, reality hits hard and fast. My life, my medical life, I should say, took a turn for the better. In a way, I came home again — back to my early American pioneer roots.

And it was a good thing I did. As you can imagine, once I questioned the orthodoxy of science, once I spoke up and said the emperor had no clothes, I was branded a medical outcast. Like most fundamentalists, my colleagues didn't take

too kindly to a different point of view —
especially one which challenged all they believed.

Well, good riddance, I say. For too long,
doctors in this country have given up their
common sense — the very thing which I believe
made this country what it is, or sadly, what it was
— for the comfort of scientific theory. No
thinking, just follow the company line. If patients
suffer, well, that's the price you pay for medical
"progress." I never understood that, and
thankfully I ran from it.

So, sometime around 1970 I came home. And
that what this book is all about — coming home.
It's a way to help you recover your common
sense and take responsibility for your own health.

Now Pm not saying every natural remedy is
viable in every case. No one in his right mind
would claim that. And *you ye* certainly heard me
say many times that certain illnesses require
specific drugs — natural remedies won't do if you
have pneumonia.

But *it's* not often, if at all, that natural
remedies can cause harm. At their best, they can
solve a problem *without* using dangerous drugs
and drug-induced side effects. At worst, they may
not work, but they usually don'! harm you.

Oftentimes, this non-invasive, non-drug
method is the first way to go. Before you spend

$50 at your doctor's office and start taking expensive drugs, try the simplest method first. The human body is a wonder. It can repair itself and usually does so without intervention. In fact, many of the results we attribute to drugs are simply the body repairing itself. The drugs have little or nothing to do with it.

So, many times, the simplest way is the best. That's what I'm offering here — simple, common-sense, tried-and-true remedies that just *may* work for you.

And remember, medicine is more an art than a science. And like art it can be fun. I'm serious about these remedies, but that doesn't mean we can't poke a little fun at Grandma and at ourselves.

Lucy died in her sleep at the age of 99 and some folks swear she'd still be alive *today* if she hadn't dipped snuff. I'm glad she didn't live to see the terrible things that have happened to her country, especially in the field of medicine.

God bless you, Dr. Lucy McDaniel Bell. I'll never forget you and the simple wisdom you instilled in a young boy's heart. I may have left it in my early years, but I came home to open arms. This one's for you!

William Campbell Douglass, MD

1

Grandma Bell's Medical Wisdom

When my Uncle John was a preteen, and already towering over *Lucy,* she would take him into the valleys of that beautiful, idyllic mountain country and send him out foraging for the right herbs. She gave him samples so that he would know what to look for. Often as not, she would reject what he brought — not fresh, too mature, not the right aroma, too bitter, not bitter enough, and on and on.

They would go early in the morning; only time to pick medicinals, she would say. Uncle John took this duty very seriously because Lucy was The Doctor and he had often seen her relieve human suffering with her concoctions. Uncle John developed a deep reverence for nature and natural healing from his boyhood experience with this gifted woman, his grandmother, my great-grandmother. Uncle John lived into his late 80s and, as far as I know, never went to a "real" doctor.

But don't get the idea Grandma Bell was a dedicated vegetarian. She used the vegetable kingdom to its fullest to defend against those Horsemen of the Apocalypse that she felt she could deal with, but she was no stranger to chicken soup, I can guarantee you. And when some neighbor was pale and puny, she told him he needed *blood,* not carrot juice. This would be in the form of rare beef, not rare pork (because of the danger of trichiasis) or rare chicken. Lucy was an acute observer and she didn't look at the eating habits of chickens everyday without noting what filthy creatures they are.

Carrot and other vegetable juices weren't known back then, because there was no technology for juicing a carrot or a cabbage. I have no doubt that she would have used these juices, where she thought them appropriate, if she had owned an Atlas Supersmasher, but there was the little problem of electricity. I don't recall Lucy *ever* having electricity in her "clinic," which was her home. How in the world did she live to be so old with no vegetable juicer, no exercise equipment for "work outs," no vitamin pills, and an outside privy?

One reason, I suspect, is that Lucy and her compatriots had a different kind of stress than we face today. They had stress all right, but it was more of a combat with nature (not counting the Great War of Northern Aggression, of course). I've used her privy at seven on a dark morning in January — I always worried about a copperhead or a spider biting me where a boy wouldn't want to be bitten, but the only thing I ever saw down there was an occasional frog. The country form of stress was more natural, it seems to me.

Heart attacks were unknown in those days, yet they ate a diet that would make a nutritionist with the American Heart Association recoil in horror. Thomas Wolfe, in his accurate portrayal of Lucy's world in the novel, *Look Homeward, Angel,* tells us what folks ate in those days:

> In the morning they rose in a house pungent with breakfast cookery, and they sat at a smoking table loaded with brains and eggs, ham, hot biscuit, fried apples seething in their gummed syrups, honey, golden butter, fried steak, scalding coffee.... At the midday meal, they ate

heavily: a huge hot roast of beef, fat
buttered lima beans.... At night they
might eat fried steak, hot squares of grits
fried in egg and butter, pork chops, fish,
young fried chicken.

I remember it well, because my Grandma
Lena Bell Williams carried on the Lucy Bell
tradition. I never missed a meal there, if I could
help it. If I would be going light on the ham she
would say, "Don't you love ham any more?" I
would correct her: "Grandma, you aren't
supposed to *love* foods — you *like* them." (Yes, I
was a smart-ass kid.)

Thomas Wolfe mentions fruits, of course,
but I want you to get a feel for all those foods
they ate that we roundly condemn today. Yet,
people just died of old age, not heart attacks,
assuming they didn't get killed from a farm
accident. Farms were dangerous places in those
days; still are, in fact.

But things weren't perfect before radio,
sterilized milk, and that contraption which
enabled people to hurdle through the air and
get to Birmingham faster than you could ride a
good horse to Jasper (a few miles north and up
hill from Ball Ground). A vast number of
children missed the joys of childhood, and the
bittersweet experience of young adulthood, by

being swept away in the constant and relentless wars of bacterial invaders.

The invaders — tuberculosis, diphtheria, tetanus, pneumonia, typhoid, even malaria along the southern coast — usually won and Lucy could only pray (she knew when to refer a case to a specialist) and do her best to relieve suffering, transmit her warmth and love by gently pressing her knurled, but warm hands on the area that hurt, and secretly decry her lack of knowledge. There was no arrogance in Lucy; she was not a faculty trained "physician;" she was only a dedicated healer, graduated from nature's university in the blue-green mountains and valleys of north Georgia.

When I knew Lucy, I was many years away from being a doctor and, in fact, never dreamed I would be one. I had such an awe for the medical profession that I just didn't think I was good enough, even though I had three generations of doctors behind me on my father's side. Lucy Bell, my mother's grandmother, didn't count with me then. After all, she wasn't university trained — what could she know?

Doctor Bill and Grandma Bell

I practiced medicine for 20 years before I came to the realization that most doctors were in it for the money, the glamour, and the sex (there weren't many female doctors back then and a doctor was considered a prince of the realm — he could have almost any woman he wanted). But after 20 years of frustration from "treating" patients with drugs that didn't work and witnessing a lot of unnecessary surgery, I thought about my long-dead great-grandmother Bell, whose great heart must have been awfully cramped in that tiny body. At age 40, I suddenly felt guilty for not having paid more attention to her and a remorse for some great healing secrets that were lost forever. Uncle John taught me what he had learned, which was considerable, but, as he would say, "I'm not Lucy"

As I became a "born-again doctor," it wasn't so much that I believed in Lucy's remedies as a realization that most of the drug therapy was useless and highly dangerous. It dawned upon me that the drugs were getting a lot of credit that they didn[5]! deserve, and that the drug companies were getting rich primarily on what I began to call a "reverse placebo effect." Many patients reasoned thusly: "the drug is making me feel terrible, therefore it is 'working' and, although I feel worse than before I started the drug, I am actually better." What was really happening was that the body was healing itself, *despite* the drugs being taken.

Then I went to another level in my conversion: Even if some, or even most, of Lucy Bell's natural remedies were ineffective from a scientific standpoint, *wasn't it better to use safe, time-tested placebos than dangerous chemical ones?* Dr. Benjamin Rush, a signer of the Declaration of Independence *and a medical school professor,* was notorious in his time for killing patients with his mercury concoctions. Lucy was a lot better doctor than that.

I too practiced a fraudulent type of medicine for many years. I didn't poison people with deadly mercury, but in the long run, I did the same thing using "modern" drugs. That is, until the weight of evidence and the weight on my heart forced me to question the wisdom of treating signs and symptoms with chemicals promoted by salesmen who knew a lot less about medicine than Grandma Bell.

The Foundations of Health

There are a lot of reasons for the march of folly, as we witness the inexorable drive to turn American medicine into an institution as "efficient" as the postal system. I will take up that subject in a separate book. What *we're* concerned with here is what you can do to protect yourself from this impersonal, expensive, and unsuccessful medical care.

The most important thing for you is to *avoid* treatment and stay healthy. And the best way to stay healthy is to follow certain principles of health. You need to adopt your own preventive medicine plan. Most doctors know little about preventive medicine and consider it more boring than watching paint dry. Grandma Bell understood the importance of prevention and I'm sure you do too.

Remember that it's not in the best interest of the drug companies or doctors for you to maintain good health. Not that most doctors actually try to make you sick, of course. Most of them are perfectly sincere and well-meaning. But there's always that little nagging fear that some technological breakthrough will put them out of business. What if, for instance, the emerging light therapy works as well for treating internal diseases as its proponents say it will? If it proves out, you will see a lot of doctors standing at busy intersections holding a sign that says: "Former Doctor - Will Work for Food."

So read on for some doctor-dodging techniques and save the doctor visit for another day. But don't be foolish. If you are not responding to herbal treatments or other natural remedies, and you do have a problem, get checked by a qualified doctor who is also knowledgeable (or at least sympathetic) in the field of natural medicine. If he says everything is okay (that is, you don't have a serious disease), then try some other natural approach, such as homeopathy or color therapy. Maybe whatever you have will go away without any treatment — some ailments are like that. Lucy said, toward the end of her life, that the automobile in some ways was the worst thing that ever happened to both doctors and patients: They make it too easy to see each other!

Wisdom Demonstrated

Grandma had a peculiar brilliance about her. She would get an inspiration, right off the wall, when under great stress to save a patient, especially a child. One time, she was called in the dead of winter with three feet of snow on the ground, to see a five-year-old child with severe, near terminal, asthma. He was blue and sweaty. It was apparent that he was losing consciousness and Lucy knew that this signified impending death. What to do? What to do? She stared at the child and rubbed her lips. Uncle John told me the story:

"She rubbed her lips nervously - she always did that in a crisis - stared at the child and suddenly turned to me: Go to the ice cream parlor bang on the door and tell Clarence you want a bucket of crushed ice - hurry! Jacob hasn't got much time to wait.'

"I skedaddled through the snow like the devil was after me, got Clarence out of bed, grabbed the ice as quickly as he had it in a bucket and dashed back to the Jacobson house. I couldn't imagine what Grandma was going to doing to do with that ice. There was plenty of snow outside so why ice?

"By the time I returned, she had an oilcloth placed under the dying boy whose eyes cried for help. Lucy grabbed the bucket and, to everyone's amazement, poured the ice on Jacob's chest. His mouth opened in an attempt to cry out but there was only a little squeak.

"Almost in the snap of a finger, I could see his pupils enlarge and he let out a long breath. In 10 minutes he was in a deep and peaceful sleep.

"As we were walking back to Lucy's cabin, I asked her: Grandma, why did you have me go for ice when there was plenty of snow just outside the door?'

"'Well,' she said, 'I wasn't sure I wanted to do what I did. I had to get my courage up and I needed time to pray. Jacob was as good as gone and I wanted the Good Lord to have time to perform a miracle.'"

With all due respect to *God*, I think He got a little help from Lucy McDaniel Bell on that cold night.

From the standpoint of modern science, Lucy probably caused a massive release of Adrenalin internally - the dilated pupils are evidence to support that presumption. The Adrenalin would cause the constricted bronchial tubes to relax and thus dilate, so the lethal chain of oxygen starvation, which causes constriction, and the constriction then causes more hypoxia, was broken.

Maybe it was Adrenalin and maybe it wasn't. Lucy Bell was a genius with a lion's heart who worked by kerosene lamp with hot compresses, plants, a certain air of omniscience, at least in front of the patients to give them confidence in her poultices and concoctions - and those old knurled, but warm hands.

Grandma Bell's Pharmacopeia included several herbal potions and poultices. She grew up in the mountains of North Georgia and lived there all of her life. She knew her surroundings and knew which herbs were helpful and which were deadly. She was a professional. Lucy also imported some herbs in dried form from the "far north," places like Cincinnati and Chicago. (She didn't like Yankees, but she would deal with them if she had to.)

Just Do It, Naturally

Today the conventional wisdom is that anything "natural" is good; anything unnatural is bad. That may be true, in general, but it certainly isn't valid across the board. Today's most vociferous herbalists will claim that herbs can cure anything and everything, and that they offer no potential for danger. After all, they're natural.

Mushrooms are natural, but eat the wrong ones and you'll be soon pushing up mushrooms yourself, along with the traditional daisies. Or try some peyote — it's natural, and you'll get to take a lovely LSD-like trip. Only one problem: it's a trip from which you might never come back.

Recently a small Japanese village was experiencing an outbreak of throat cancer among its older people. Doctors looked for the cause of this extremely high cancer rate that was very localized in this one village.

They found the culprit. These old villagers used a certain herb once a week as a tonic. They'd been doing it for years. One small problem: the herb contained a known carcinogen. After a decade or two of use, the herb was causing throat cancer in almost all who had been taking it. So much for the safety of "*all* natural."

2

Grandma Bell's Favorite Herbal Remedies

It's with a bit of reluctance that I include the following list of herbs and their potential uses. Grandma Bell kept much of herbal expertise in her head and it died with her. I don't claim to have her herbal knowledge; I'm not Lucy, either. But I do know that herbalists have a long tradition of healing the sick — even during those times when traditional medicine had nothing to offer. It is an ancient and vast Pharmacopeia and what follows will merely be scratching the surface.

Remember: Like nutritional supplements, and indeed like drugs themselves, these traditional herbal remedies do not work for everyone. And before you try any of these remedies, *be sure you note which are for internal use,* and which are meant solely for external application. We will indicate when an herb is not to be taken internally, but even with those recommended for internal use, always start with a small dose and watch for signs of toxicity (nausea, vomiting, headache, depression, joint pain, stomach ache, blurred vision, diarrhea, palpitations etc.) and for allergic symptoms (skin rash, difficulty breathing, joint pain).

Preparing Medicinal Herbs

To use herbal remedies effectively, you must know how to properly prepare poultices, teas, tinctures, and infusions.

A *tea* is made by simply boiling (actually the water should be just *below* a hard boil, since boiling allows valuable volatile oils to escape in the steam) the leafy parts of the plant and the flowers for your treatment. Again, if you are trying something new, *use caution.* Start with a small dose and work your way up. Watch for vexatious symptoms, such as those described above.

When the tea is brewed for 15 minutes to several hours, the tea is called an *infusion.* The biggest problem with teas and infusions is that they only use the part of the plant that is water-soluble. With some plants that's all you want, but many plants have properties that can be used better in other ways. Remember that these are biological preparations, so they can spoil or develop fungi. Keep them refrigerated and don't keep them any longer than you would any other food, such as milk or tomatoes. As with any other food or preparation, the fresher the infusion, the better. I wouldn't keep them around for more than a day or two.

A *decoction* is a more vigorous extraction of a plant's properties than an infusion and is used for roots, barks, twigs, and some berries. Add one ounce of dried herb to one pint of cold water and simmer for thirty minutes to one hour. Strain and store the liquid in a cool place. The standard dosage is one-half cup three times a day.

A *tincture* is a highly concentrated variety of an infusion, but is made with alcohol instead of water. The dose is usually several drops to one tablespoon. Take the whole bottle and your eyes may pop out. To make a tincture, place the herb in a large jar and cover it with brandy, vodka, or gin. Seal the jar and store it in a cool dry spot for two weeks, shaking it occasionally. At the end of the two weeks, strain off the liquid into another clean dark bottle for storage. Some herbalists recommend that you send the herb through a wine press to squeeze out all the juice.

A *poultice* is any soft and moist mass applied *hot to the surface of the body. Sometimes* oatmeal or flour is mixed with the mass to make a paste. Many claim that the only therapeutic effect from a poultice, at least as far as any internal benefit is concerned, such as the use of a poultice over an inflamed gall bladder, is in the heat. In most circumstances, I think they are right, but not in all cases.

A *compress* is made by soaking a towel in a hot (180 degrees) herb tea and applying it to the affected area. Wring out the towel before applying it and replace it after it no longer feels warm. Keep the area under compress for up to 30 minutes.

Grandma's Herbs

So, with the above information in hand, the next time you or a loved one is "feeling poorly," give one of the following a try.

ALOE VERA

Use for:
burns, cuts, snake bites,
gastrointestinal problems

This herb is related to the lilly, but you would never know it to look at it. Grandma Bell used to make a tincture with the root of this plant to treat colic and as an antidote to the rattlesnake's bite. In fact, the plant was known as the rattlesnake's master. If you happen to get bit by a rattlesnake, I don't suggest you rely solely on the aloe plant. You can use the gel (I wouldn't take the time to make a tincture) to treat the wound, but get to a doctor as fast as you can.

You can grow aloe very easily in a window pot and you will be glad you did if you get a burn or cut. The "leaves" are more like knife blades with a thorn on the end and make a great addition to the family plant collection. Growing an aloe vera plant in your home is a great way to have a first-aid kit handy for treating burns. For burns and cuts, take one of the lower leaves, cut it lengthwise and squeeze out the gel. Apply it directly to the injured area. The gel acts as a disinfectant and anaesthetic (the relief from pain is almost instantaneous) and helps restore the skins natural pigmentation. Externally, the gel may be used liberally as needed.

Another reason Grandma kept an aloe plant around was because it works wonderfully well for many gastrointestinal problems. She used it to treat habitual constipation, especially for persons with sedentary habits.

Back in the late 1800s, a tincture of aloe was indicated for amenorrhea and was said to be highly effective. Even today, the herb is being recommended for many other ailments including asthma, colds, convulsions, hemorrhages, and ulcers. But because there's no money to be made by the drug companies, very few, if any, scientific studies have been done to support the use of aloe in these conditions. Personally, I don't think it would hurt to try, especially if you start out with low dosages.

If you want to use the fresh aloe plant internally there are a few things that you need to know. If you're pregnant, stay away from any internal use of aloe. The same goes for children and the elderly because this herb can cause severe intestinal pain. But if you are a healthy adult, take up to one tablespoon of aloe juice or gel three times daily.

The preferred way to take aloe internally is in capsule form. You can buy these at your local health food store and the dosage is one capsule, up to three time daily. Be warned: many products on the market today contain very low amounts of aloe. Make sure the product you buy lists aloe as the first or second ingredient on the label.

AMERICAN HELLEBORE

Use for:
rashes, sores, lice

American hellebore was not very plentiful in the mountains of Georgia, but when Grandma Bell was able to find it, she new what to do with it. This herb can be very deadly if it is not used properly, but Grandma Bell found that it worked wonderfully for rashes and sores. After slicing the rhizome (stem), she would boil it with vinegar and apply the fluid to the affected area. She also brushed a strong decoction of it through the hair to kill lice — a big problem in Georgia.

The Russians place this herb in their vodka and claim that it helps reduce the pain of sciatica and rheumatism. Hellebore is used in several hypertension drugs because it lowers blood pressure and slows the heart rate. Homeopaths use it for fever, flu, headaches, and measles.

Because this herb is so toxic, I don't recommend that you try to use it as a home remedy. One false step and you could be six feet under — and we don't want that. In fact, Grandma's most popular use for American hellebore was to poison the birds that ravaged the farmers' crops.

ANGELICA

Use for:
chronic bronchitis, rheumatism,
gout, fever, digestive problems

This was once the herb of choice for the 16th-century English. It was used for just about everything — from rabies to flatulence — and if you carried a piece of the root in your pocket it would serve as a preventive against witches and the evil eye.

Grandma used the root for more practical matters, such as bronchitis and fever. Today it is used to treat digestive diseases, including gastritis and indigestion. Angelica root is best administered in the dose of one or two teaspoonfuls of an infusion made with an ounce of the root to a pint of water, or of white wine.

'For external use, you can preserve angelica in honey to make an excellent tonic. It has also been applied in a strong decoction for rheumatic and gouty joints. *A quick word of warning: this herb may contain a possible carcinogen, so don't use it more than you have to.*

ANISE

.

Use for:
indigestion, flatulence,
bronchial problems

Since Roman times it has been used as a digestive aid. It's the herb that imparts the licorice flavor to candy. Hippocrates recommended anise for clearing the respiratory passages.

Many of the farmers around Grandma Bell used anise seeds to treat their flatulence. It was a flavorful remedy that consisted of one tablespoonful each of anise seed and honey in a glass of water and simmered for 15 minutes.

The action is in the seeds which can be purchased in health food stores or you can grow the herb yourself and collect the seeds in late summer. To make a tea, crush a teaspoonful of seeds for every cup of boiling water and let steep for twenty minutes. Three cups a day will give you the maximum benefit. If you have purchased an anise *tincture,* remember that it is much more concentrated and you only need one-half teaspoon in your cup of boiling water.

This is one of those herbs that would make Grandma Bell stand back and laugh at modern medicine, because it is just now realizing what she knew 100 years ago. Grandma Bell often made an infusion with the bruised seeds and gave it to nursing mothers to help them produce more milk. Auburn University recently reported that cows sprayed with anise oil were able to produce more milk than cows sprayed with other fragrances. Don't ask me how Grandma figured this one out, but she knew.

Anise can cause nausea and/or diarrhea. If this occurs, discontinue until the symptoms clear and then start again with a smaller dose. *Avoid during pregnancy.* In fact most herbs, as with conventional drugs, should be avoided during pregnancy.

ARNICA

Use for:

heals wounds, skin irritations, rheumatism, blood tonic

If you thought lard was only good for cooking food, think again. Grandma loved to cook arnica flowers in lard and rub the ointment on sore muscles and joints as well as sprains and bruises.

This same ointment can also be used to reduce the swelling of inflamed breasts. Simply rub the ointment gently on the affected part. This treatment is not recommended for nursing mothers.

In the 1980s, German researchers found that arnica did indeed contain chemical compounds which reduce inflammation. Arnica flowers should only be used externally as they can be deadly if taken internally.

However, Grandma often made a tea from the arnica *root*, yarrow, and St. John's wort that proved to be extremely effective in combating phlebitis, thrombosis, varicose veins, and ulcerated legs that many nursing mothers experience.

BARBERRY

Use for:
arthritis, gout, cancer,
sore throat, nerves, diarrhea

Not to be confused with bayberry (see below). In Grandma's day, barberry was used for quite a few problems. You can gargle with a mixture of water and barberry for sore throats. It also has some astringent properties. Best of all, this herb is safe, so you can try it for yourself without worry.

Barberry is a liver stimulant and, therefore, has been known to be effective for many types of liver disorders. Grandma used barberry to treat cancer, because cancer patients always suffer from liver problems. Obviously, it wasn't a cure for cancer, but stimulating the liver did help improve the patient's condition.

Going through some literature about barberry, I found that many people like to make remedial preserves out of this highly nutritious berry. And I can hardly blame them as the barberry is absolutely delicious. Dr. H.C.A. Vogel had the best recipe for barberry preserves in his book *The Nature Doctor,* because it sought to preserve the vitamin content by using raw berries.

His recipe is as follows:

"Put the freshly picked and fully ripe barberries through the mincer. Then squeeze the pulp through a sieve. The pips and skins will remain in the sieve and you will have the clean puree and juice. Add 100 g (3 oz) of raw cane sugar to 500 g (1 Ib) of barberry puree and stir well. When the sugar has dissolved, add 200 g (7 oz) of honey and finally 200-250 g (7-8 oz) of thick grape sugar syrup. Stir the mixture until well blended. If the mixture is too thin, add a little more raw cane sugar. Then, pour into glass jars as you would with jam."

Once the berries are preserved, you can eat them whenever you have problems with diarrhea. Or just eat it on your toast for breakfast, if you want.

This recipe is a great way to preserve the berries for the winter, but I prefer to eat the berries right off the branch. You know how much I hate sugar, especially when it comes to treating health problems.

BAY

Use for:
rheumatism and other pains,
bladder infections

With the leaves of the bay tree, Grandma would make a decoction that would reduce the sting of insect bites. She also used the root bark in a decoction to treat bladder infections and other diseases of the urinary organs.

Another external application that Grandma used was to cook the leaves in lard and apply the ointment to sore muscles and joints. It also eased the pain of rheumatism, bruises, and many other pains.

BAYBERRY

Use for:

sore throat, fever, scrapes, insect bites, varicose veins, hemorrhoids

Once the darling of herbalists, this fruit of the laurel tree is now a suspected carcinogen. But then again, everything is a suspected carcinogen in today's world. This was one of Grandma Bell's favorite herbs, but that was mostly because of its pleasant fragrance.

But it did have medicinal uses. Grandma used a bayberry poultice to help heal scrapes, insect bites, and cuts. She also rubbed it on varicose veins and hemorrhoids to relieve the swelling and discomfort.

Today, you can buy bayberry in capsule form from your local health food store. I don't recommend that you take more than one capsule three times daily as you need it, because large doses of this herb can induce vomiting.

BIRCH

Use for:
bladder and kidney ailments, rheumatism

Indians used it to relieve headaches and fevers. American settlers soon learned the value of Birch — not the least of which was as a switch for disobedient children. I can tell you from personal experience that Grandma knew that treatment.

Birch, like willow bark, contains a compound related to aspirin; thus it has analgesic properties. The best way to use birch for medicinal properties is to make a tea from the leaves. Drinking two or three cups of tea daily, between meals and for at least four weeks has eased the pain of rheumatism and gout. The tea is also good for bladder and kidney ailments.

Grandma loved to use the sap of the birch to treat what she called "scaly diseases of the skin" or psoriasis. She also found that the sap was effective on scurvy and intermittent fevers.

About the only time I remember thinking Grandma Bell was losing it was when she treated her neighbor who was suffering terribly from rheumatism. Grandma had made a bed of fresh birch leaves and asked her friend to lie down in the middle of it. After lying there for a while, the neighbor broke into a profuse sweat. I wasn't able to hang around to see if it worked, but Grandma insisted her friend was as "fine as frog's hair." But Grandma said that about a lot of things.

Lucy never ceased to amaze me as to the number of things she could do with a birch tree. Apparently, the Indians she learned from used the birch tree for everything from building canoes to treating many of their aches and pains. One of her more interesting remedies was for the *itch*. After reducing the bark to a pulp, she would mix in black powder (not modern gunpowder — there's a big difference!) and cream. She said this was good for treating enlarged glands as well.

BLACK ALDER

Use for:
fever,, diarrhea, sprains, ulcers,
canker sores, sore throat

Lucy said that this American species of alder is both "astringent and diuretic" which I tend to doubt, since diuretics are seldom astringent. However, its astringency resides in the leaves, as well as in the bark, with both of which a decoction is prepared for the treatment of diarrhea, blood in the urine, and intermittent fever. A decoction of the bark, when bruised, can be applied to contusions, sprains, and ulcers. It is also effective as a gargle for a sore throat and as a mouthwash for canker sores.

Lucy would often use the bruised leaves as a breast application to lessen the secretion of milk or dissipate indurations during lactation. She also used it to treat hives. The decoction she made was with half an ounce of powdered bark to a pint of water, taken several (three or four) times a day.

BLACKBERRY

Use for:
sore throat, kidney problems

Rubus fructicosus, or blackberry, is unusual in that practically any part of the plant can be used for medicinal purposes — the bark, the leaves, the root, dried blackberry powder and even the fresh blackberries. Sore throats respond well to an infusion of hot wine and blackberry leaves.

Grandma used blackberry root to treat infantile diarrhea and what she called "summer complaint" diarrhea. She generally administered it in a decoction made with water or with milk, an ounce in a pint and a half of liquid being boiled down to a pint.

In the spring, Grandma would send Uncle John out to collect blackberry branches that were just beginning to bud with new leaves. She would use the new shoots to make a wonderful spring tea. She claimed it was good for the kidneys. The tea was very simple to make. She would pour boiling water over the young leaves and flowers and sweeten it to taste with a touch of honey. This was one of my mother's favorites.

BLACK MUSTARD

Use for:

coughs, colds, headaches, sinus congestion

Probably 99 percent of our readers have never heard of this herbal remedy, but Lucy Bell considered it one of the most important. Black mustard is for external use and is perhaps the best herb in the world for poultices.

It is recommended that the poultice be applied *to the feet,* no matter what part of your body is crying for succor. Make a foot bath of a tablespoonful, or more, of dried black mustard to hot water. The theory is that the blood will flow away from areas of congestion and to the feet. This works well for coughs, colds, headaches, and sinus congestion.

If you want to *increase* the circulation to an affected part, such as a skin infection, then apply a black mustard poultice directly over the infected area. A paste works best in these cases: one tablespoon of black mustard to four tablespoons of flower. Add enough water to make a paste that can be applied to a linen or other convenient tissue, and applied to the skin of the affected area.

The use of mustard plaster can be painful, because if it's left on too long, the skin will blister.

As an irritant, mustard is renown — just ask any of the "doughboys" (if you can find one) who were subjected to mustard gas attacks in World War I. Therefore, I advise you to place a piece of gauze between the plaster and the body, to prevent the plaster from adhering to the skin. It should be applied from ten minutes to an hour, according to the degree of its action. If blisters or sores begin to form, discontinue using the plaster and apply a poultice of grated carrots to the sores.

BLADDER WRACK

Use for:
sprains, arthritis, obesity

This is a fascinating herb that you have seen hundreds or thousands of times, but probably gave little attention. It's the common seaweed found on beaches all over the world. It's the one with the fronds and the little "bladders" all along the fronds. Hence the term bladder. ("Wrack" means marine vegetation.) Grandma never made it to the sea in her life, but had she made it, you can bet she would have brought back a bucket full of dried bladder wrack.

A popular 19th century method of bladder wrack poultice is tried and true for sprains and arthritis: Wash thoroughly; cut into short pieces about the length of a string bean, *leaving the bladders intact.* Cover with water, vodka, rum, or whatever your spouse is drinking too much of (tell him it's for a good cause) and seal the bottle for a week to ten days. Apply it directly or as a poultice in soaked toweling or any convenient cloth.

Bladder wrack has been recommended as a treatment for obesity because it has a diuretic effect when taken internally. I do not recommend this therapy for the overweight for two reasons:

(1) Diuretics do not work for obesity. The problem is *fat*, not water, and any weight loss will be only temporary.

(2) It is the most God-awful, slimy mixture that you can possibly imagine and, even if you were starving, I doubt that you could drink it. It's available in health food stores, but I do not recommend taking it internally until it has been proven to have some practical use thereby.

BONESET

Use for:
arthritis, common cold, flu

Boneset has been used for centuries by American Indians and Europeans. A hot infusion is a popular and efficient remedy in the forming stage of muscular rheumatism, sore throat, bronchitis, and even influenza. It earned its name from its power of relieving pain in the limbs during bouts with influenza.

This herb can be taken as a tea and is recommended by herbalists for everything from arthritis to colds. Boneset is famous for its ability to promote sweating which makes it especially effective against a cold or flu virus.

I remember one particular instance when my Uncle John was sick in bed with a terrible fever and sore throat. I thought this was going to be a great opportunity to see Grandma at work. But to my utter disappointment, Grandma simply covered him with several blankets and gave him a cup of hot tea.

I knew there had to be something else she could do for my uncle, so I asked, "What else does he need?"

I was hoping she would send me out to the woods to get some special herb that only she knew about, but instead, she replied in that soft but confident voice, "Nothing for now."

I was beginning to get restless, and Grandma could tell that I was expecting some fireworks. Graciously, she continued. "All he needs for now is a hot cup of boneset tea and a warm place to rest."

Uncle John slept for most of the day, but anytime he would wake, Grandma was quick to give him another cup of tea. I noticed that while he slept Uncle John would perspire heavily. I thought it was because of all the blankets (and they were partially responsible), but Grandma Bell told me later that boneset tea "makes ya sweat," which helped break Uncle John's fever.

The next day, Uncle John was feeling much better. He still had a bit of a sore throat, but the fever was gone and he was able to get back to work. I don't know for sure what part the boneset tea played in his well-being, but Grandma used it, so it must do something.

Grandma's recipe for boneset tea was really quite simple. It consisted of one teaspoon of boneset and an equal amount of peppermint added to one cup of boiling water. She would then cover the cup and let the herbs steep. After about ten minutes she would strain the tea and add the juice of half a lemon. Boneset is a bitter herb, so I recommend that you add two teaspoons of honey.

CATNIP

Use for:

flatulent colic, toothaches, bronchitis, diarrhea, cramps

Grandma's main use for catnip was for the relief of flatulent colic in infants, but she also used it to promote menstruation when it was retarded or painful. Once used as a sedative for cramps and upset stomach, catnip tea does seem to have some calming effects. And Grandma used it locally to help with toothaches and other local pains. Many people still use it as a nightcap to help them sleep. I wish it did for women what it does for cats.

Catnip is best taken in an infusion made with half an ounce to an ounce in a pint of water, and in the dose of from a teaspoonful (or less, for infants) to a tablespoonful. You can make a tea by pouring boiling water over the dried leaves. Use more of the leaves than you would for ordinary tea and be ready to cover your cup. Catnip's aroma can be rough on the sinuses.

CAYENNE PEPPER

Use for:
fever, hemorrhoids, motion sickness,
sore throat

This is one of those herbs about which so many claims are made that it's hard to separate reality from myth. Cayenne pepper contains capsicum, a known stimulant which can also be applied externally for painful joints. Many claim it works as an internal detoxifier. Many also say that drinking it in water is a sure way to stop a cold from taking hold. *Use sparingly — too much cayenne pepper taken internally can cause kidney damage.*

Because there are so many outrageous claims made about cayenne pepper, I'm just going to give you the things I know Grandma Bell used it for. Grandma didn't know that cayenne pepper stimulates the stomach to produce gastric acid, but she did know that it helped a "feeble stomach" (that's indigestion to you modern folk).

In fact, modern medicine usually prescribes a bland diet for heartburn and indigestion because it is generally considered nutritionally incorrect for people with gastrointestinal problems to heartily season their food. But Grandma knew better.

Later we'll talk extensively about the positive effects garlic can have on the entire body, and especially the circulatory system. While cayenne pepper is not the anti-infection agent that garlic is, the spice is extremely effective in reducing the strain on the heart and circulatory system.

Mannfried Pahlow, author of *Healing Plants*, says "Spicy seasonings in particular intensify the progress of almost all vital processes, which results in increased vitality. If you want an all-around feeling of well-being, frequently add spicy seasonings like paprika, cayenne pepper, ginger, mustard, or turmeric to your foods....

"In Mexico, where people enjoy eating fiery chili peppers, and in the Balkans, where hot paprika is popular, fewer people suffer heart attacks than in this country. As research over time has revealed, the spices used are partially responsible."

Grandma didn't have the luxury of knowing facts like this to back up what she did, but she knew that the body needed a "jump start" every now and then. I can still remember the charge she got when I first bit into her "mild" chili. It nearly sent me through the roof and she laughed about it for days. Pll tell you one thing, it got my heart beating.

Lucy also used cayenne pepper and other herbs of the same nature to prevent or relieve motion sickness. And for treating the sore throat often seen in serious illnesses like scarlet fever and diphtheria, Grandma knew that no application was so efficient as a strong gargle or wash made with cayenne pepper.

Capsicum comes in many varieties, from Africa to the American south. Cayenne is considered the best of the capsicums for therapeutic uses and is very popular as a cold remedy. Take one teaspoon each of cayenne and sea salt, grind them together into a paste, add a cup of boiling water and, after the mixture has cooled, a cup of vinegar. Take a teaspoonful every half hour. This same mixture can also be used as a poultice or a gargle.

CHAMOMILE

Use for:
indigestion, cramps, insomnia,
insect repellant, pain reliever

Chamomile is a pretty flower, somewhat like a daisy, that grows in the meadows, another of God's tiny wonders. You can grow it at home, but it's not the same as the wild form, it doesn't even look the same.

Grandma never went anywhere without carrying some chamomile. It has a variety of properties which have been proven effective. It is an anti-inflammatory, and works in cases of indigestion and menstrual cramping. The tea is a calmative, and makes a great nightcap, especially for fussy children.

In fact, chamomile is the pediatric herb of choice, according to Doctor/Professor Grandma Lucy Bell. It's safe — that's always the first consideration with *real* doctors like Lucy — and it's effective in a wide range of illnesses. It works for indigestion and clears up infant diarrhea. Ointments can be made to treat various minor skin irritations and as an insect repellent. The sedative action of chamomile is almost as good as a teaspoon of vodka. (You'd be surprised how much alcohol there is in medicines.)

Externally, Grandma made fomentations by saturating chamomile flowers with hot water, or hot vinegar and water, which would form a soothing application for local pains including toothaches, earaches, abscesses, sprains, and the like.

CHAPARRAL

Use for:
bad breath, infection, cuts, bruises

The local Indians taught Grandma everything she knew about this herb. It was known as the stink weed with the pretty name and it tastes like something out of a creosote factory.

Ironically, it's good for bad breath. I guess it asphyxiates every bug in your mouth. A study reported in the *Journal of Dental Research* reported that chaparral mouthwash reduced tooth decay by 75 percent. I don't know that this is true, but it is possible, considering the herb helps the body ward off infection.

Many claim it's a cure for cancer — I have a hard time believing this one, too. However, I do know that Grandma used it very effectively to treat external wounds. People with kidney disease should avoid chaparral.

CINNAMON

Use for:
diarrhea, vomiting, poor digestion

Current research confirms what older herbalists have known for some time — cinnamon works to kill various fungi and bacteria — including the microorganism which causes botulism and certain staph infections. Grandma also used it to relieve vomiting.

You can take cinnamon in a number of ways, but it tastes the best with your pumpkin pie or in hot apple cider. An infusion may be made with the bruised bark in half a pint of boiling water, and administered in doses of a tablespoonful or two every hour. If you like to use cinnamon oil, be careful because it can burn your tongue.

CLOVES

Use for:
toothache, vomiting, colic

Cloves used to be considered an aphrodisiac, but are more suitable for allaying vomiting and promoting digestion. Grandma's favorite use for cloves was to ease the pain of a toothache. She had the patient roll the clove around in his mouth, "bruise" it gently by chewing and, with his tongue, press it against the sore tooth. It is a mild anesthetic and has germicidal properties.

Bruised clove tea can be used as a sedative. As can a teaspoonful of clove oil added to a glass of hot water. Make the tea by infusing bruised cloves in half a pint of boiling water. Grandma used tablespoonful doses of the tea to help colic.

COMFREY

Use for:
bruises, sores, athlete's foot

Used by Grandma as a poultice for severe bruises and sores. When I asked her where she learned how to use this one, she said that it had been passed down from "ancient times." That was her way of saying, "I'm not going to tell you." And who am I to argue, as long as it works.

Today we know comfrey contains allantoin which is used in numerous over-the-counter ointments to help speed healing of skin problems. Some claim external use can cure athlete's foot.

This is an herb that is great for soothing the skin. Lucy often used it to treat fissures of the nipple or chafed nipples by applying a hollow section of the fresh root over the sore organ. There are many commercial comfrey salves on the market that are recommended for nursing mothers. However, mothers must be careful not to let their infants ingest any comfrey, so I don't recommend that you use the commercial products. Grandma's method is probably the safest, and I would wash thoroughly before allowing your infant to nurse. Grandma said her method would work for other skin problems, as well.

Do not take it internally. When taken internally, comfrey is not comfy.

COD-LIVER OIL

Use for:

*arthritis, gout, eczema, psoriasis,
high blood pressure*

Grandma Bell, and every grandmother, great grandmother, and mother I knew when I was growing up, believed that cod liver oil was the most important supplement, "tonic," and "restorer" in the world. They were right. I don't know how they knew it; they just knew.

Since the early 1800s and before, cod-liver oil has been used as a popular remedy for chronic gout and rheumatism. Also, the oil has been used successfully both internally and topically for the treatment of chronic eczema and psoriasis.

In addition, cod liver oil, high in the omega-3 oils:

  * Thins the blood
  * Increases mental alertness
  * Protects the arteries from damage
  * Protects the kidneys
  * Reduces the blood triglycerides
  * Is antiasthmatic
  * Lowers blood pressure
  * Is cancer-preventive
  * Reduces the risk of heart attacks and strokes

* Is anti-inflammatory
* Is effective in the treatment of rheumatoid arthritis
* Helps in the treatment of migraine headaches

Cod-liver oil is an excellent anticoagulant and can be used in place of Coumadin, *which may induce osteoporosis.* It is high in vitamin D content and, whereas I have often decried the use of vitamin D as a supplement because of the overuse of this hormone in our foods as an "enrichment" in a natural product, such as cod liver oil, I cannot recommend it with enough enthusiasm. It is a superb nutrient and has even been found to be of use in the treatment of multiple sclerosis. *{Medical Hypotheses,* 21(2) :1986)

The average dose of cod-liver oil is a tablespoonful three times a day, an hour or two after meals. It is better to begin with half or a third this quantity. You can get too much of anything and tolerance to cod liver oil may vary. Because of its high vitamin A and D content, get a liver function test every six months if you are taking large doses (more than a tablespoonful per day).

COLTSFOOT

Use for:
bronchitis, coughing

This difficult-to-kill nuisance weed has a leaf shaped like the hoof of a horse. It's excellent for coughs in an infusion and can even be smoked. I didn't say you *should* smoke it; I said you *could*. When mixed with other herbs — rosemary, thyme, chamomile, and others — Grandma found that smoking coltsfoot was very effective for pulmonary affections (especially chronic bronchitis). She argued that smoking was the only effective way to use coltsfoot. Use a pipe.

When I was a preteen, living in Ball Ground, we used to smoke "rabbit tobacco" out behind the barn. It was a sickly grey weed. I have no idea what it was, but it had a pleasant aroma. We used old newspapers for the wrapping. Again, not something I would recommend.

I happen to disagree with Grandma on this one, because in my book, smoking is just not an option for treating disease, except in rare instances. Instead, I recommend that you administer coltsfoot in a decoction or infusion made with an ounce of the dried leaves and flowers to a pint of water. I think you'll find these effective.

DANDELION

Use for:
liver disorders, gall bladder disease,
jaundice, warts

Dandelion is said to be good for a "sluggish liver." Trouble is, I don't know how to diagnose a sluggish liver. It sounds like a bad thing to have, but I don't know what it is — and Grandma isn't here to explain it to me.

I suspect the diagnosis was used much like the modern medical experts when we invoke "a virus" when we don't know what's going on. That's OK though. Patients want a *diagnosis'*, it makes them feel better. (We have a saying: "The name of the game is the name.") Try it for your "sluggish liver" — let me know if it helps. Grandma said it works and she was usually right.

The leaf is usually used as a tea for many ailments including gall bladder disease. It must be picked when young otherwise it is extremely bitter. But for the "sluggish liver/' use the *root*. Dandelion tea is also said to be good for colds, diabetes, tuberculosis, rheumatism, and arthritis. Simmer two ounces of the sliced root in two pints of water. Boil it down to one pint. Drink a half glass two or three times a day. Or you can take two to four fluid ounces of a decoction each day.

The roots can also be made into a caffeine free coffee that works well for insomnia and digestive problems. First, roast the roots until they're brown and hard. Then grind them into a powder and brew like regular coffee.

If you have warts, the dandelion may move from the most hated weed in your yard to the most beloved. Inside the stem of the dandelion is a milky substance that dries up warts quicker than any commercial product. Simply squeeze the stem until the "milk" exudes and apply it to the wart. Let the milk dry and *dont* wash it off. When it has disappeared, apply it again. Do this religiously and your warts should start turning black and falling off in three or four days.

ECHINACEA

Use for:
colds, measles, arthritis, malaria

This one of the great herbs with plenty of research to back it up. This purple cornflower was an important part of Lucy's armamentarium. European research has revealed a natural antibiotic in echinacea called echinacoside which works similar to penicillin. But it has a broader spectrum than penicillin in that it will attack viruses and fungi as well as.bacteria. It also has an ability to fight radiation side effects (Grandma didn't know about that part).

Echinacea has even gotten the endorsement of a university pharmacologist. Dr. Varro E. Tyier, professor of pharmacology at Purdue University, says that echinacea can ward off colds. I think it's better than vitamin C in this regard. Lucy thought so too, but of course, she didn't *have* vitamin C.

Groups as disparate as the American Indians and the Chinese swear by echinacea. In the 1800s, it was used for measles and other childhood diseases, arthritis, and malaria. It is said to be one of the best herbal "blood purifiers" and it may act as a stimulant to the immune system. Echinacea works as a mild antibiotic.

Take the root and boil it, then simmer for 10 minutes. A half cup, cut up, is enough, in a half pint of water. Drink a cupful three times a day. Commercial preparations are also available, but fresh is always best.

ELDER

Use for:
coughs, bronchitis

Grandma Bell knew what she was doing when it came to herbs, but even she was wary of using elderberry — except in jams and jellies. She used to form a syrup by boiling the juice from the berries with crabapple juice and a little sugar to treat coughs and bronchitis.

The berries are harmless, but the seeds, leaves, and stems can be deadly. And don't eat the berries until they have been cooked. Elderberry contains a substance that releases cyanide — the deadly poison. If you want to use elder, I suggest you try Grandma's syrup or purchase commercial elderberry tea and stir in some honey to treat your cough.

EUCALYPTUS

Use for:
ulcers, gangrene, colds, bronchitis

It was very difficult for Grandma to get her hands on eucalyptus leaves or oil, but when she did she found that it worked especially well on stomach ulcers and gangrene. The powerful oil derived from eucalyptus has many medicinal properties. You're certainly familiar with its ability to unstuff clogged noses, but it also has antiseptic and astringent qualities. Grandma used it in a poultice for healing many types of skin ailments. Inhaled with steam, the oil offers relief to the symptoms of bronchitis and croup. It is an excellent expectorant.

EVENING PRIMROSE

Use for:
arthritis, rashes, diarrhea,
asthma, general pain

The oil of evening primrose seems to help some women with premenstrual syndrome, but definitely not all of them. It may also be helpful in the treatment of cystic breast disease. EPO has shown great promise in the treatment of arthritis, but there are conflicting studies from Finland that *theoretically* show EPO will make arthritis worse. However, *clinically* most studies have shown that evening primrose oil helps most arthritics. I'm like Grandma Bell: go with what helps the patients and leave the theory to the professors.

Grandma's journals indicate that evening primrose works effectively on "infantile eruptions" (various skin rashes). She said, "It is advised that about the flowering season, the small twigs with the bark of the large branches and stem, retaining their leaves, should be dried in the shade. Of these a strong decoction is made, with which the eruptions should be bathed several times a day.... I have also used it in diarrhea and in asthma."

FENUGREEK

Use for:
constipation, fever, ulcers, boils

Another herbal cure all, fenugreek has been used for centuries, and with some success. It seems to work well as an expectorant, a stomachic, and a febrifuge. Folk remedies suggest fenugreek for its laxative abilities and as an aid in curing ulcers. Medical research has partially confirmed these abilities.

Externally, you can pulverize enough seeds to make a paste when mixed with eight ounces of water. The paste soothes boils and wounds.

FEVERFEW

Use for:
headaches, toothaches, rheumatism

This is a daisy, but not the regular daisy. You can grow them, but the product is available in health food stores. It doesn't do much for fevers, as the name would imply, but this is an herb with definite therapeutic value. Granny grew it and used it for headaches. She didn't know about serotonin inhibitors, but that's what makes the herb remarkably effective for headache, including the migraine variety. It will not cure migraine headaches, but will contain it as long as the feverfew is continued. Fortunately, the herb is quite safe and can be taken for long periods of time without danger *unless* you are taking a blood-thinning medication. Then it should be avoided.

Grandma liked to use a decoction or an infusion of the herb. She used these much like she did chamomile, to allay the pain of local inflammation like toothaches or rheumatism.

GARLIC

Use for:
bronchitic, heart disease, meningitis,
etc., etc., etc.

Vampires hate it; Gilroy, California loves it ("The Garlic Capital of the World"). Hippocrates prescribed it for intestinal parasites, Albert Schweitzer used it as an antiseptic in the African bush, and for four thousand years it has been used as an amulet against the evil eye. When I first started my travels around the world in the 1960s, I was surprised to see in Third World countries that most babies had a garlic bud on a string tied around the neck.

And I think the Roman naturalist, Pliny, went a little overboard in claiming 61 uses for the herb, including the cure of leprosy, asthma, and epilepsy and, he said, it was a great scorpion repellant. (If you try that one, let me know.) I love garlic and you probably love it, too. Even Russians, who have the blandest diet in the world, love garlic. Gastronomy would not be nearly as sweet without the "stinking rose" and, in Gilroy, if you say something stinky about garlic they will just sniff at you, or worse, breathe on you.

Even budding babies are high on garlic. A study reported in the *New England Journal of Medicine* found that babies drink more breast milk when it tastes of garlic.

Dr. Robert Hermes must have gotten wind of this because he has devised a new material composed of garlic and plastic that will coat artificial heart valves, thus taking advantage of garlic's anti-clotting and bacteria-fighting abilities. The two dreaded complications of heart valve replacement are infection around the new valve and blood clots which can cause a fatal stroke.

Dr. Hermes said: "If it sounds like garlic is a wonder drug, well, it *has* been the wonder drug of traditional medicine for 2,000 years. Finally, Western science is taking a hard look at garlic and finding that all those generations of folk healers were on to something." (Granny would be self-effacing, but definitely pleased.)

When I read that investigators in communist China had cured some cases of meningitis with garlic, I was, naturally, very skeptical (you know how commies lie). But when I read that researchers in New Mexico had achieved similar results, I investigated further on the Chinese claims. What they had done was give the garlic *intravenously* to their meningitis patients! What a great idea — you'd get hanged for trying that in this country. I might, however, try the procedure at my African clinic. African doctors are willing to try anything that sounds reasonable and, for all they care, you can spear the FDA.

There are two true wonder drugs: one is penicillin and the other is garlic — and garlic, in the long run, may prove to be the superior one. It was here first, and while penicillin is losing its potency, garlic isn't. Besides, garlic will do things that penicillin can't do.

No one ever claimed that penicillin would cure or prevent cancer, but there is mounting evidence that garlic will not only prevent but cure some malignancies. In both Italy and China, it has been found that high garlic intake correlates with a decreased incidence of stomach cancer. Animal and laboratory studies clearly indicate that garlic will prevent and/or control malignant melanoma, one of our fastest-growing and most deadly forms of cancer.

Dr. Ben Lau, perhaps the most experienced garlic investigator in the world, is so enthusiastic about garlic as a preventive of cancer that he has suggested putting it in peanut butter, just like we put iodine in salt to prevent goiter. Like salt, which conies iodized and uniodized (some people are allergic to iodine), you could buy your peanut butter garliced or ungarliced.

Garlic, like so many other herbs, has remarkable effects on triglycerides and cholesterol. While the cholesterol level is poorly correlated with heart disease, the triglyceride level does correlate well. Garlic lowers both. It also inhibits "platelet aggregation," the sticking together of these little blood cells, which leads to clot formation.

Doctors at Tagore Medical College in India did a study on garlic and its effect on coronary artery disease. Their findings were quite remarkable. They fed garlic to 222 patients with coronary artery disease (CAD) and compared them with a control group of 210 CAD patients who did not receive garlic. The death rate in the garlic-consumers was reduced by 50 percent in the second year of the study and 66 percent in the third year. Second heart attacks were reduced by 30 percent in the second year and by 60 percent in the third year. Cholesterol and blood pressure readings were also lowered in the garlic-fed group.

The Wistar Institute in Philadelphia has found garlic to be effective in reducing low-density lipoprotein, the one that correlates with heart disease, and to increase high-density lipoprotein which is protective against CAD. So don't take aspirin for your heart — you don't have an aspirin deficiency — take garlic (and cod liver oil).

Of all the marvelous attributes for garlic, one seldom mentioned or known about is its attributes in the treatment of arthritis. Lucy said this herbal treatment came from Devon, England, as far as she knew, and she swore by it.

Skin the cloves of four large heads of garlic (there are about six cloves to a head so you will have 24 cloves) and marinate them in 500 ml of brandy (French cognac is considered best, but your medicine will be more costly) for about ten days.

Take a teaspoonful of the marinade (actually a tincture) diluted in a half glass of water first thing every morning.

Two questions often come up regarding garlic:

(1) Should garlic be taken in its natural form or is the capsule just as effective? and

(2) If taken naturally, should it be raw or cooked? It appears that any form of garlic, raw or cooked, natural or capsule, seems to be effective.

Wouldn't you think cardiologists would be rushing to get their patients on garlic? The doctors aren't rushing, but their patients are — garlic sales are up astronomically all over the world and Japanese Kyolic and German Kwai are in a titanic battle for the garlic market — may they both win.

Grandma said, "Bruised cloves of garlic and poultices of boiled onion are admirable remedies for chronic bronchitis in children. They should be applied over the whole front of the chest. Internally, garlic is a very useful agent in the same affliction."

I recommend eating one clove of garlic per day (or its equivalent in commercial tablets), more if you feel an illness coming on.

GINGER

Use for:
indigestion, nausea, motion sickness, arthritis

Grandma used it to ease that "feeble stomach" and to stop flatulence. She also swore by its ability to stimulate circulation. Ginger is an excellent seasick remedy — start taking it before you get on board.

During Lucy's day, ginger root was the treatment of choice for nausea. Motion sickness was not much of a problem up in the hills, because nobody went anywhere, but it is effective for motion sickness and works better than the popular drug, Dramamine. I have always said the only reason Dramamine worked was because it had such a dramatic name.

According to doctors from Odense University, Denmark, 75 percent of arthritics are given relief from the use of ginger, both in pain and swelling. There are no side effects from it and the FDA can't ban ginger from the marketplace.

For the scientists among our readers, ginger inhibits prostaglandin and leukotriene synthesis.

Ginger root, taken in capsules or as a tea, is very efficacious for heartburn and, like its use in motion sickness, is better than the expensive commercial products.

I like my ginger pickled, the way they serve it at sushie bars. I eat it by the handful. Many people don't particularly like it. You can probably find encapsulated powdered ginger at your health food store. An amount equivalent to two teaspoonfuls daily will be enough — more is better.

GINSENG

Use for:
indigestion, vomiting, nervous disorders

This is a tricky one. I don't know if Grannie used it, but she probably did. If there is any herb considered to be a cure-all, ginseng is it. I wonder if there is a Chinese living who doesn't take ginseng — I doubt it.

The trouble with ginseng is that it's hard to prove anything, because the root varies so in potency and different types of ginseng have different compounds in them.

Ginseng is said to be an aphrodisiac (which it isn't). It is used as a pick-me-up, an aid to memory, for coughs and colds, to raise blood pressure, to *lower* blood pressure and as a tranquilizer. How can it be a stimulant and a tranquilizer at the same time? How can it raise the blood pressure in those who are *hypotensive* and lower it in those who are *hypertensive'*?

Orientals have an artistic and mystical approach to herbal medicine. They explain these apparent contradictions with the ancient Doctrine of Signatures: the healing herb resembles the part of the body it cures. So, as ginseng has a vague resemblance to the whole body, it can do just about anything, depending on what you need. I have a little difficulty accepting that but you can believe it if you want — it'll work better (and presumably in the right direction) — if you do believe it.

On a more scientific level, ginseng contains saponins which some scientists call "adaptogens" meaning they can normalize things. This could explain the apparent contradictions mentioned above — the adaptogens bring the body to a state of homeostasis, meaning balance. But its hard to measure effectiveness as the concentration of saponin varies greatly, even in roots from the same area. The Siberian ginseng is said to be the most consistent in its action and to have fewer side effects. Pregnant women, children, and people with hypertension should avoid ginseng.

GOLDENSEAL

Use for:
sore gums, hemorrhoids, colds, flu,
constipation, infections

There are so many contraindications to the use of this compound that I hesitate to recommend it at all. Although I have my doubts, some tree-huggers like Jethro Kloss, author of *Back to Eden*, call it "one of the most wonderful remedies in the entire herb kingdom — a real cure-all"

It is recommended for sore gums. Massage your gums with it, using your finger. The bitter tea of goldenseal can be taken internally and, according to one author, will "combat internal infection, aid digestion, cleanse the body after an infection, and even help hemorrhoids." I'm not sure I believe such catholic claims for this little tea, but it does have certain proven ingredients, such as berberine, that inhibit the bacteria that cause diarrhea.

You can make the tea in the usual manner using a teaspoonful of the powdered root to a cup of boiling water — steep ten minutes; drink two or three cups a day.

But there is a down side with the use of goldenseal: You should be pretty healthy to use it otherwise you can do yourself considerable harm. If you have had a stroke, have high blood pressure or heart disease, or suffer from glaucoma or diabetes, don't take this herb.

If used in excess, goldenseal can cause nausea, vomiting, and — more serious — depression of your white blood cell count.

While Uncle John said he could spot goldenseal under a shade tree from 50 yards away (it has a hairy purplish stem with yellow-brown bark, leaves that look like raspberry, and in the spring it has greenish-white flowers and orange berries), Lucy didn't collect much of it and used it judicially. She said: "You'd better be healthy or this herb will make you unhealthy."

GOTU KOLA

Use for:
psoriasis and other skin conditions

Gotu is a leaf, not related to the kola nut with which it is sometimes confused. It's called a brain food and a life extender. Some herbalists use it topically for wrinkles, psoriasis, and other skin conditions. None of this has been proven, but I like the name.

I was surprised to find that gotu isn't listed in the *National Dispensatory of Herbals,* an official government publication, published in 1879. Uncle John told me Granny had never mentioned gotu kola, although it is popular today. I found out why: first, gotu kola is cultivated only in China and India and, second, it simply wasn't known in the West until after World War II.

HAWTHORN

Use for:

*heart palpitations, high blood pressure,
irregular heart beats*

This herb is another example of the remarkable wisdom of the ancients, including Grandma Bell, in the treatment of disease. Since researching this monograph, my respect for Lucy and all her forebears has increased immensely.

Hawthorn is a classic cardiovascular drug in its natural form. Angina-, the terrible, crushing pain of an oxygen-starved heart, can be relieved by this herb. It rates right up there with the digitalis leaf (night shade) as a heart and blood vessel therapeutic agent. But it has, sadly, gone the way of most natural remedies and most cardiologists have never heard of it. Hawthorn is effective in palpitations, high blood pressure, and irregular heart beats. But, as with many natural remedies, you must be patient; it doesn't act almost instantly as do some drugs.

Dr. Varro Tyier, professor of pharmacology, Perdue University, is convinced that hawthorn is a stimulant to the heart and has a definite place in the treatment of heart disease. It is certainly nothing new that this herb has cardiac effects. American settlers of the 18th century used hawthorn for the treatment of angina pectoris, the agonizing pain of an oxygen-starved heart. (This was not coronary artery disease but arterial *spasm* as coronary arterial disease was rare in the 1700s.) They also took it for high blood pressure.

It has now been proven that hawthorn dilates the blood vessels of the heart and thus relieves angina. For heart rhythm disturbances, such as atrial fibrillation, it can also be effective if used faithfully over a long period of time. Herbal remedies often take time and patience. If you expect overnight results, in most cases, you will be disappointed. The quick-fix mentality of our culture has hurt the reputation of herbal remedies.

Make a tea from two teaspoons of the crushed hawthorn leaves in a cup of boiling water. Steep for 10 minutes and add honey and lemon for taste. Two or three cups a day will do.

If you have heart disease, and are taking prescription drugs, don't go hog-wild on me and stop your medication for this or any other herb. *Sudden discontinuance of prescription cardiovascular drugs can be fatal.* I don't want you haunting me in a courtroom — or from heaven for that matter.

HONEY

Use for:

*wounds, gastroenteritis, chafed nipples,
diarrhea, etc.*

When Grandma Bell started her country practice, refined sugar was a product of the future and honey was the primary form of sweetening. However, honey was used for many things other than a sweetener.

Since the time of the ancient Egyptians, honey has been a medicinal of great importance, especially for the treatment of wounds. Although Dr. Jarvis, in his bestselling book, *Folk Medicine*, goes overboard in crediting honey with the power to cure many diseases, everything from sinusitis to bed wetting, there is no doubt that honey has unique properties and Lucy took full advantage of it.

Honey taken by mouth is very effective in the treatment of gastroenteritis and it was Lucy's first line of defense against this common childhood disease. And for nursing mothers, it is probably the best treatment for chafed nipples. It will soothe the pain and promote healing, but is completely safe for the infant.

In her journals, Grandma wrote, "It may be mentioned that propolis, a resinous exudation with which bees cover the bottom of their hives, is reported to be beneficial in the treatment of acute and chronic diarrhea."

The best type of honey to use is unprocessed, of course. You may not be able to buy it at your local grocery store, so contact a local bee keeper or stop at one of those road-side stands and buy the freshest honey you can find.

HOPS

Use for:
rheumatism, toothache, colic, bruises

The main use for hops today is in the manufacture of beer — and that takes a *lot* of hops. Before hops were discovered, people drank mead, a fermented malt, sweetened with honey and flavored with herbs. But hops brought about a revolution in drinking with the introduction of beer which now finances football, baseball, and a lot of similar noble pursuits.

People turned to the new intoxicant with such gusto that a movement was started in England to ban hops because the taste was so wonderful "it would enslave the people." That was 400 years ago. They lost and the people have become enslaved to the hop — but no one seems to mind.

The Brits can't cook, but they sure can brew a good beer — 400 years of practice helps. They have always taken brewing very seriously. Back in the old days of the 17th century, you would receive a severe penalty, such as a term in prison without beer, if you, as a manufacturer, "sophisticated" your product, i.e., added sugar to the mixture.

According to herbal experts, an infusion of an ounce of hops to a pint of boiling water, taken a glass-full before meals, will cure "debility," lack of appetite, and "nerve trouble." Seems to me a cool Guiness stout would do the same thing without all that trouble. Pm not trying to drive you to drink, understand; it's just a semi-scientific observation.

Grandma used hops externally to relieve the pain of muscular rheumatism, abscesses, spasms, toothache, colic, and bruises. For these problems, Grandma would place the strobiles into a bag and moisten them with hot water, vinegar, or alcohol, and apply them to the painful part.

For internal use, Grandma insisted that the best preparation is the infusion, but she also knew the benefits of a good beer: "A pure and strongly hopped beer contains all the virtues oi this agent (the infusion)." She used hops internally for an irritable bladder and other affections attended with genito-urinary irritation.

There is absolutely no doubt that hops will induce sleep. A lot of people who have taken "an infusion of hops" before driving can attest to that. Simmer a quart of water containing an ounce of hops down to half the volume and then strain it. Take an eight-ounce glass of this infusion at bed time. But then, *there's* always the Guiness....

HOREHOUND

Use for:
sore throat, coughs, bronchitis, indigestion

This interesting herb with the naughty name and the bitter taste has been used for centuries as a sore throat remedy, for chest congestion, and the ancient Greeks used it to treat the bite of mad dogs — for rabies (I wouldn't rely on that if I were you).

Horehound has been used in commercial cough syrups for a hundred years or more, but the FDA is removing it because they say horehound has not been proven to be of benefit to you, the *stupid* consumer. The FDA hasn't been of much benefit, either.

Lucy used horehound as a stomachic tonic in indigestion and in chronic bronchitis to restrain secretion. It has also been used in chronic rheumatism and, like other bitter herbs, in intermittent fever.

An infusion made with an ounce of horehound in a pint of hot water may be given in doses of a wineglassful. The expressed juice should be administered with honey or milk, in the dose of a teaspoonful or two several times a day.

JUNIPER

Use for:

rheumatism, week stomach and appetite, arthritis

Grandma used it in a poultice to help ease arthritis pain. She also had gout and rheumatism patients eat the berries. She didn't know they worked because they helped the elimination of uric acid — she just knew they worked. I remember going over the Grandma's house and noticing a muslin bag that always hung over her bathtub. She said it was a bag of juniper needles that helped her rheumatism.

Juniper works well to soothe tired muscles. The next time you come home from work tired and worn out, stick your feet in a hot herbal foot bath made with juniper needles and notice the difference in how you feel. Grandma used to tell her farmer friends to do this. Don't boil the needles, just pour the boiling water over them and wait till it cools to a comfortable temperature. The hotter the better.

If you have a week stomach or appetite, Grandma would tell you to eat juniper berries every morning before breakfast. She had an interesting dosage: one berry the first day, two the second, three the third, on up to fifteen or sixteen. Then reduce the amount the same way until you get back to taking one a day. I don't know if it does any good, but you might try it.

Juniper was once used as a diuretic, but it isn't always safe, because the kidneys may be sensitive to it. Personally, I would forget about using juniper internally.

KELP

Use for:

asthma, indigestion, constipation,
emphysema, bronchitis

Granny had heard of seaweed, but I doubt she ever saw any. She never left Cherokee County except for a trip to Atlanta about once a year. Big cities like Atlanta, population 100,000, had little appeal to country folks — too many fancy people and neurotic horses. It was unsettling to the nervous system.

Lucy would have appreciated kelp, a contemporary name for seaweed, if she would have had access to it. After all, according to folklore, it cured just about everything: asthma, indigestion, constipation, emphysema, bronchitis, urinary problems, obesity, colitis, ulcers, gall stones, arthritis, nervousness, skin diseases, and insect bites. Let's see, what's left? Oh yes, it cures cancer and is antiatherogenic.

But in spite of this broad spectrum claim to near-perfection, there is actually a lot of scientific evidence that kelp is indeed a marvelous nutrient. Most of the research has been done in Japan, but Jane Teas, a highly respected researcher in

America, has done a lot of work on kelp in the treatment and prevention of cancer.

A little seaweed in your diet won't hurt; Lucy would have approved. (Also see Bladder Wrack in this chapter.)

LAVENDER OIL

Use for:
indigestion, cancer, local pains

This is another hoped-for cure for cancer. Work on animals has been phenomenally encouraging, especially for breast cancer. When animals with cancer of the breast are fed lavender oil, 60 to 70 percent of the cancers disappeared! Human studies will begin next year in England.

Grandma used lavender tea as a remedy for indigestion and as a mild tranquilizer. The infusion is said, when too freely taken, to occasion colic.

Fomentations made with lavender enclosed in bags allay local pains, like other plants of the labiate family.

LECITHIN

Use for:

cirrhosis

I know you're not a drunkard but perhaps you have a friend who is. Alcohol researcher Charles Lieber of Mount Sinai School of Medicine reports that lecithin, a soy bean extract, can prevent heavy drinkers from developing cirrhosis of the liver. Cirrhosis is usually what does alcoholics in, unless they stumble in front of a speeding beer truck.

Dr. Lieber fed the human equivalent of eight cans of beer a day to baboons (they had a great time and didn't want to discontinue the experiment) over a ten-year period. A portion of the baboons was also fed three tablespoons of soy lecithin a day. None of the simians on the lecithin supplement developed cirrhosis. But seven out of nine of those not given the lecithin supplement developed severe cirrhosis. Soybeans are not the only source of lecithin. Peanuts, poppy seeds, and dandelion flowers are also rich in lecithin. Great-grandma Bell knew about the therapeutic efficacy of dandelion. A hundred years ago she was using it for "disorders of the bile" — right on target again, Grandma.

LEEK

Use for:
digestive stimulant

Grandma liked to use the leek in many of the same ways she used garlic, with one exception:

You've swallowed one of those giant paper clips? — and it's attached to your garage door key? Oh boy, have you got trouble. Not if you were in Grandma Bell's neighborhood. No problem. First, she would say, don't panic, everything is going to be fine. Lucy would quickly boil up a mess of leeks and have you eat them, and *nothing else,* for 24 hours. The fibers of the leek will encase the metal objects in a nice sheathe and the missile will be delivered back into the outside world painlessly and effortlessly. (Don't forget to recover your garage door key.)

But some problems are too difficult even for the leek remedy. In Ball, Indonesia, 24-year-old Sudarsana went to the hospital complaining of stomach pains. X-rays revealed a picture of a junk shop. The incredulous doctors operated and found in the stomach a key hanger, a bamboo meat skewer, two kitchen knives, a butter slicer, a tablespoon, and a fork.

A spokesman for the hospital said it was possible Sudarsana had swallowed the objects while not of sound mind. Seems possible. (Ref: Sapa-Reuters, *The Citizen* (South Africa), 2/6/94)

LEMON BALM

Use for:

upset stomachy colic, gas, stress, insomnia, fever

During Grandma's -day, balm tea was a popular and refreshing drink, when made with the fresh plant, and taken cold. The hot infusion of the dried plant is one of the mildest that can be used to favor the operation of diaphoretic (sweat-producing) medicines. This helps cool the body and often helps break a fever.

Grandma used lemon balm as her premiere sedative; perhaps the smell itself had a calming effect. In the 17th and 18th centuries, lemon balm was used to calm and soothe the nerves and impart a general feeling of well-being. Culpepper, the famous herbalist from that time period, had this to say about lemon balm: "Let a syrup made with the juice of it and sugar ... be kept in every gentle woman's house to relieve the weak stomachs and sick bodies of their poor and sickly neighbors."

LICORICE

Use for:
ulcers, coughs, bronchitis,
congestion, constipation

Granny used licorice to treat ulcers. If she was treating serious "indigestion" and bleeding commenced, she knew there was trouble. Then she would throw the book at them: cayenne pepper, licorice, pure cream, aloe vera root, and no doubt other things I never knew about and are now forgotten.

A powdered, concentrated form of licorice has also been found to be very effective against canker sores in the mouth. It is still used as a chief component in herbal cough remedies and cough drops. For children, take a decoction made with one teaspoon of the root in a cup of water. As a powder, it has been used as a laxative.

MARIGOLD

Use for:

cancer, ulcers, wounds,
amenorrhea, contusions

The marigold is used for the treatment of inflammation and as an antiseptic. This is one flower that Grandma may have been a little too proud of because she insisted that it possessed stimulant and resolutive virtues, and used it to treat congestions of the liver, jaundice, amenorrhea, scrofula, and. even in typhoid febrile states.

She also employed marigold internally and externally in the treatment of cancer, because she said it disposed cancerous ulcers to heal. A solution of the extract and a decoction of the herb were used for this purpose. I'm not sure whether or not this is true, but I don't think it would hurt to try. I haven't seen any studies indicating one way or the other.

A saturated tincture of the flowers is said to promote the cure of contusions, wounds, and simple ulcers. You can also simmer the flowers in water, milk, or apple cider vinegar. Use this mixture cold for inflammation. When it has drawn in the heat to the poultice, exchange it for another cold one.

MARSHMALLOW

Use for:
infected wounds, skin inflammations,
sore throat

Until I started researching this book I had no idea that marshmallow was an herbal remedy with an honored past. I didn't even know it was a plant. I doubt that the marshmallow air puffs some people eat have much to do with the herb except for the flavor. (Lucy said it was just candy with a marshmallow flavor.) The marshmallow root is dried and powdered for poultices. It's an old remedy for infected wounds and skin inflammations. The whole root can also be chewed as a sore throat remedy and the French give the whole root to teething children. It's also a good laxative and "stimulates the kidneys."

MEADOWSWEET

Use for:

arthritis, fever, respiratory problems

Lucy knew about this herb, but it is seldom mentioned in today's natural healing books. That's puzzling because it was the forerunner of aspirin. Lucy used it for arthritis, fevers, and respiratory problems. She didn't know that it contained salicin, a cousin to aspirin, she just knew that it worked. Unlike valerian, meadowsweet smells really nice and was used by our unwashed ancestors, who lived in close proximity to their farm animals, to give an almond scent to the house.

Make a tea from the dried herb and drink one cup every day. However, a word of caution must be given: meadowsweet shouldn't be given to children with colds or other viral infections because of the danger of Reye's syndrome.

THE MINT FAMILY

Use for:

*indigestion, colic, headache, diarrhea,
heart palpitations*

The sultry days of a Georgia summer were pure misery for many people before the advent of air conditioning. The hot, wet air followed you everywhere; there was no escape from it. Well, almost no escape. Grandma had a recipe that made the days seem like a splash in the local stream.

The streams running through the mountains of Georgia are wonderful for trout fishing, something my Uncle John loved to do. The water is sparkling clean and, best of all, cool. Feeding into these streams are natural springs that produce the coldest and best tasting water in the hills. Grandma took advantage of these springs whenever she could and used the water in many of her remedies. She had a spring that wasn't too far from her home and loved to make a refreshing drink in the summertime heat with its water. Her recipe was about as simple as they come: twist or squeeze one cup of mint leaves into a half gallon container and then fill with cool spring water. Strain and serve. It did wonders for a boy who couldn't drink enough water in the heat of July. We drank a lot of iced tea, too.

But what Grandma didn't tell me was that the mint was helping my body. I guess she knew little boys don't like things that are good for them — something about parental wisdom. But somehow I don't think that would have stopped me from drinking her mint water.

There are several types of mint, including peppermint, spearmint, and the European pennyroyal, that can usually be used inter- changeably. However, peppermint is generally regarded as the most effective of the group.

The name peppermint describes the sharp, biting taste of this plant, whose odor, when fresh, is likewise very powerful, but refreshing. In the mouth it produces a pungent sensation, followed by a sense of coolness and numbness, increased by inhaling strongly. When swallowed, it produces a diffusive warmth in the abdomen.

From almost the beginning of time, peppermint has been used as a digestive aid. And today, scientific studies have shown that it increases the flow of bile. It also works to calm the muscles of the digestive system, which helps calm an upset stomach.

Lucy swore by peppermint, in the form of tea, as a treatment for indigestion. A hundred years later, research done at Purdue University proved her to be right. The tea is good for indigestion, headaches, and asthma (inhaled as a mist).

Menthol comes from peppermint and is widely used in commercial products for chest congestion and joint pain or "rheumatism." Peppermint oil will often give relief from toothache and a small amount, ten drops, mixed in water is effective in childhood diarrhea. Grandma recommended it to relieve menstrual cramps.

The bruised fresh leaves of peppermint have been used to allay colic, headache, and other local pains. A hot infusion, given in tablespoonful doses, is commonly employed to relieve diarrhea, vomiting, flatulence, indigestion, and other abdominal pains. There are also several commercial teas on the market that are both medicinal and great tasting.

Spearmint is a much milder form of medicine than peppermint, but can be used for most of the same maladies with the same preparations. However, because it does have a milder nature, spearmint is generally preferred for infantile cases. Be sure and check with your pediatrician before giving any herb to your child.

ONION

Use for:
high blood pressure, infections

The onion contains many of the same medicinal values as garlic, but with smaller doses of the antibacterial and antifungal components. That means that, like garlic, onion has hundreds of uses — many of which medical science is just beginning to investigate. Grandma didn't usually use the onion to treat specific ailments, but used it more as a general "wellness" food. She new that garlic was a more potent healer, but when I was sick, I did notice the number of onions I consumed went up dramatically.

Onions also help protect the heart, and are now being used to lower the "bad" cholesterol. In addition, recent research has shown that onion increases HDL, the so-called "good" cholesterol.

It has also been touted as a natural way to lower blood pressure. Many scientific experiments have shown that raw onions will have a lowering effect on mildly high blood pressure. One experiment, in fact, found that rats injected with an onion extract had significantly lower blood pressure than those in the control group.

PARSLEY

Use for:
urinary problems, high blood pressure,
bad breath, gonorrhea

Men were embarrassed to talk to Lucy about their sex life or about any problems with their plumbing. But when she would get a question from the wife concerning her husband's urinary problem, the patient would get two consultations for the price of one. Lucy would recommend that she make up a tea from parsley greens — the stronger the better — and have him drink it often. She also recommended a lot of watermelon to keep the urine flowing which will prevent bladder infection.

But men were not the only beneficiaries of parsley tea. Grandma often used the modern garnish to treat uterine disorders like amenorrhea, "scanty" menstruation, and dysmenorrhea.

Freshly bruised parsley leaves were a popular remedy that Grandma used for any enlarged external glands. She also used the dried leaves and the juice to cure gonorrhea, periodic fevers, and neuralgia; but the seeds are said to be superior to either in the treatment of intermittent fever, when given in the form of a recently prepared and strong decoction. (Don't count on it to cure your gonorrhea — Lucy wasn't perfect.)

PASSION FLOWER

Use for:

stress, insomnia, neuralgia, piles, burns

At one time people would smoke passion flower to get high. It does have some tranquilizing effect and continues to be used by herbalists to relieve tension and help fight insomnia. Some European sedatives use passion flower. Passion flower tea is one way to experience its calming abilities. With all these soporific attributes, why is it called passion flower?

The passion flower indigenous to our Southern states was used with extraordinary success during Grandma's early years to treat tetanus and neuralgic affections. The root was used in the form of an extract as an application for the initial lesions of syphilis, irritable piles, and recent burns. Grandma prepared the herb as an extract by evaporating to dryness the expressed juice of the leaves gathered in May, and was given in the form of powder, and in the dose of from one to four teaspoonfuls.

PIPSISSEWA

Use for:

rheumatism, urinary disorders, fever, diarrhea

Grandma swore that this was the best diuretic available, and she used it to help those with kidney problems. The American Indians and early settlers used it to treat typhus (unsuccessfully), as well as rheumatism and kidney disorders. The former disease in the joints was treated with fomentations or poultices of the leaves, while a hot decoction of them was administered internally to the production of sweating. Because of this latter characteristic, it has also been prescribed for intermittent fever.

In cases of scanty or suppressed secretion of urine, Grandma often resorted to pipsissewa. Sometimes she would even use the decoction to treat diarrhea.

PSYLLIUM

Use for:

constipation, diarrhea, hemorrhoids,
heart disease, ulcers

It's not pronounced "pee silly um" but "silly urn" as the T' is silent. It's a remarkable herb in that it is good for both diarrhea and constipation. It's the outside coating of the seed that gives it such remarkable properties. As it comes in contact with water, the mucilage in the coating swells and turns into . a jellylike substance. Regularity can usually be achieved by taking a teaspoonful of the seeds two or three times a day — it has an unpleasant texture, but maybe you can get used to it. *Be sure to take plenty of water* when taking psyllium or you might explode from constipation.

In recent years, psyllium has become highly touted as a preventive against heart disease. This is probably due to its effectiveness on the digestive system — the place where most heart problems begin.

PUMPKIN SEED

Use for:
tapeworm, prostate

This is one of *my* favorites, although it may not be used very much today. Maybe you can try it on your dog, but be sure to check with your vet first. He'll probably think you're crazy, but at least you asked.

According to Grandma Bell, pumpkin seeds are among the most efficient remedies for tapeworm. To treat this horrible problem, Grandma would take from one to two ounces of fresh pumpkin seeds and peel them of their "outer envelope." She would then beat them into a paste with finely powdered sugar and dilute it with water or milk. Three or four hours after drinking the mixture, she would follow it with one or two tablespoonfuls of castor oil. Before taking the medicine, the patient should fast for 24 hours.

The oil from the pumpkin seed has shown promise in improving the condition of the prostate. Some claim that prostate problems can be worsened by the presence of parasitic worms in the lower intestine. Pumpkin seed oil kills these worms.

RED CLOVER

Use for:
cancer, eczema, stress, coughs

This little flower is said to have anticancer properties. I was skeptical until I learned that studies at the National Cancer Institute identified *four substances* in red clover that work against cancer. Red clover is also a good source of vitamin E. If you are a man, and you are taking large doses of this herb, let up if you start getting the urge to wear lipstick. There are a lot of estrogen-like substances in red clover.

Red clover is not going to cure your cancer, but because of the findings at the National Cancer Institute, maybe it's a good cancer preventive. If you want a little cancer insurance, make a tea from the dried flower tops and take it a few times a day.

Lucy never used red clover to treat cancer, but she did use it to treat eczema. She also used it as a muscle relaxer and as an expectorant.

SLIPPERY ELM

Use for:

*infections, sore throats,
coughs, indigestion*

This was one of Grandma Bell's broad spectrum remedies. She used it for practically everything — and so did the Indians. The inside of the bark is covered with a slippery, mucilaginous substance that has healing properties. It is used topically as an application for infections and as a tea, it is good for sore throats, coughs, and indigestion. You can also buy slippery elm bark lozenges to help that irritating sore throat (take one up to three times a day).

SPIRULINA

Use for:

NOTHING

This pond slime is mentioned in the hope of discouraging you from using it. It's been highly touted as a cure-all by the tabloid press. According to the promotion, it will cure everything from cancer and obesity to wrinkles.

Spirulina is high in protein, but also extremely high in iron content. And unlike most vegetable sources of iron, it is readily absorbed into the body. Many spirulina samples have been found to be contaminated with mercury and lead. Wild animals push it away before drinking out of a pond. You should do the same.

ST. JOHN'S WORT

Use for:
viral infections, wounds, ulcers, bruises, varicose veins

I don't know if it helped St. John's warts, but early Christians used it to drive out the devil. And did they have some great names for this innocent herb: "The Lord God's Wonder Plan" "The Devil's Scourge" and "The Witches Herb" and many similar. The ancients attributed to it stimulating, drying, and cleansing virtues, held it to be diuretic and emmenagogue (promotes the menstrual discharge), and a specific remedy for wounds, ulcers, and burns.

In Grandma's days it was given for the relief of chronic inflammation of the lungs, bowels, and especially the urinary passages. Grandma used it for digestion and to relieve gastritis and ulcers. Externally, she applied it in the fresh state, bruised, for contusions and for the relief of local pains. Her favorite way to use St. John's wort was to immerse the flowers in a bottle of olive oil and let it hang in the sun for a month or two. This would give the oil a dark red color and made a very popular application to excoriations, wounds, and bruises. An infusion can also be used by preparing an ounce of the plant in a pint of hot water.

Expectant mothers suffering from thrombosis, phlebitis, and varicose veins will find a tea made with St. John's wort, yarrow, and arnica root to be an excellent remedy for these troubles. This tea will also help soothe irritating hemorrhoids. The oil from St. John's wort is an excellent treatment for many skin problems and works wonderfully on dry, scaly skin.

I've found that applying the crushed leaves and flowers of St. John's wort to inflamed nerves works very well. And now researchers from New York University and the Weizman Institute of Science in Israel have found that St. John's wort has properties that curb the growth of retro viruses like AIDS.

THYME

Use for:

*sore throat, fever, headaches, bad breath,
insect repellant*

Thyme, pronounced "time" is from the mint family. Grandma liked to use thyme as a seasoning to help improve digestion. She also employed a drop or two of the oil to treat bronchitis (especially in the elderly), amenorrhea, and externally, as a stimulant application to bruises and in muscular rheumatism.

The leaves and flowers can be made into a tea in the usual way to make a bittersweet drink that is quite pleasant. It's a calming agent and helps sore throats. Making a poultice is also a great way to treat a sore throat. It's said to be a digestive aid and a fever remedy. It's also a good seasoning for many foods, but insects don't like it which makes it a good insect repellant. There are a lot of other claims for it from headache to bad breath. You can try it for these ailments. If it doesn't work, at least you will have had a nice cup of tea and you might get a pleasant therapeutic surprise.

VALERIAN

Use for:

*insomnia, muscle tension, anxiety,
stomach cramps, epilepsy*

Valerian really stinks! So much so that you would think it *has* to be good for you — and it is. This stink weed has been a cure-all throughout history. The Greeks and the Romans used it as a decongestant, pain reliever, and even as an antidote for various poisons. In the Middle Ages, it was so popular that it was dubbed "all-heal." None of its supposed magical properties have been proven, but *it's* popular in Europe as a sleeper and tranquilizer. Our ancestors, when they arrived here, were amazed to see that the American Indians were also using it as a sedative. That's pretty strong evidence to me that it works.

It has been called the "Valium of the 19th century" because of its ability to relax the body. While it has a similar effect on the body, it *isn't* related to Valium in any way. And, unlike Valium, it is not addictive and has very few unpleasant side effects.

According to Grandma's medical journals, "Valerian is not a cure for hysteria, but it is a most valuable palliative when employed to avert or mitigate hysterical paroxysms provoked by some accidental cause. Especially is this the case in females of weak constitutions and excitable temperament, and who are exhausted by care and anxiety. (No, I'm not making this up!) It is still more efficient in preventing the development of those hysteroidal attacks which weak and morbidly sensitive girls and women are liable to.... Valerian is one of the best remedies for nervous headache, ... flatulence, ... and is equally efficient in relieving infantile colic.

"Valerian is one of the innumerable articles that from time to time have been vaunted as remedies for epilepsy, and, allowing for the common error of confounding epilepsy with epileptiform reflex convulsions. And even with hysteria, there can be no doubt that, in large doses and long continued, it has sometimes cured the disease in females and young children, and especially when it originated in fright or some analogous impression. Even in these cases it must be administered in large doses and be long continued, ... to give permanent strength to the nervous system."

In the U.S., you can buy it in capsule form (take one up to three times daily), or you can make your own "home brew." I recommend the latter approach. Put two teaspoonfuls of the powdered valerian in a cup of boiling water —

steep for 15 minutes. Or place ten drops of the extract into your favorite liquid. You can disguise the disgusting taste with honey, spices, and lemon. Take too much valerian and you will get a headache, or worse.

WHITE MUSTARD

Use for:
indigestion, constipation, bronchitis,
rheumatism

In Grandma's time the mustard plaster was a tried and true remedy for chest congestion. It could be made with either white or black mustard seeds (See also BLACK MUSTARD for the recipe) and is great for arousing the central nervous system. Many also used it to ease arthritis pain.

For internal purposes, the white mustard seed is preferred over the black seed. In strong cases of indigestion with constipation, the white mustard seed has long been employed with a dose of one teaspoonful in a half-cup of water, before or after meals. This will prevent flatulence, promote digestion, and keep the bowels regular. But this treatment will lose its effects if it's used regularly.

Grandma loved to use an infusion of mustard seeds to treat the obstinate cases of hiccups. It didn't always work, but it did arrest this irritating symptom in many cases.

Many people argue that mustard is not an effective treatment for chronic bronchitis or chronic rheumatism, but Grandma knew differently. She would often make foot-baths with white mustard seeds to relieve any type of internal congestion.

Grandma often told a story of a Dr. Weber (she never gave his first name) who claimed that a hot bath made with white mustard seed was extremely effective in treating childhood pneumonia. According to her journals, he placed the child in a baby-tub filled with water at a temperature of 100-105 o F., and had the skin rubbed thoroughly until it began to look red. This process required from seven to ten minutes, then the child was wiped dry and put into a bed previously warmed. No ill effects were observed from allowing the genitals to remain unprotected. The bath might be repeated as often as every three hours. I definitely would *not* recommend this treatment instead of penicillin, but I don't think it would hurt to give it along with the medication. I also think it would probably be effective for colds, bronchitis, and rheumatism.

WILLOW

Use for:
headache, rheumatism, arthritis,
indigestion

The forerunner of aspirin, willow has many of the same medicinal attributes as aspirin. Grandma used it to relieve headache pain and reduce inflammation of joints. It also made good switches for recalcitrant children — trust me, I know.

Like simple bitters, willow bark appears to increase the appetite and improve the digestion, but if you use it extensively, it can cause constipation. A decoction or infusion may be made with an ounce of the bruised bark to a pint of water and taken three or four times a day. Grandma often used willow bark to treat intermittent fever, but I do not recommend it for this or to treat flu symptoms. Because of its similarity to aspirin, it can cause Reye's syndrome.

This is not an herb I would recommend growing in your back yard, unless you have a lot of land.

Appendix

Quick Reference Guide to Common Ailments

abscesses — see chamomile, 53; hops, 82.

amenorrhea — see aloe, 30; marigold, 92; parsley, 99; thyme, 108.

angina — see hawthorn, 78, 79.

arthritis — see bladder wrack, 44, 45; evening primrose, 64; garlic, 71; juniper, 84;

meadowsweet, 94; white mustard 111; willow, 113.

asthma — see aloe vera, 30; cod-liver oil, 57; evening primrose, 64; peppermint, 97.

athlete's foot — see comfrey, 55, 56.

bladder infections — see bay, 38; hops, 81; parsley, 99.

coughs — see black mustard, 43; coltsfoot, 59; elder, 63; licorice, 91; slippery elm, 105.

croup — see eucalyptus, 64.

diabetes — see dandelion, 61.

diarrhea — see barberry, 36, 37; black alder, 41; blackberry, 42; chamomile, 52; goldenseal, 76; honey, 80, 81; peppermint, 95, 97; pepsissewa, 101; psyllium, 102.

diphtheria — see cayenne pepper, 51.

dysmenorrhea — see parsley, 99.

earaches — see chamomile, 53.

eczema — cod-liver oil, 57; red clover, 104.

epilepsy — garlic, 68; valerian, 109, 110.

fever — see angelica, 32; bayberry, 38; black alder, 41; boneset, 46, 47; cayenne pepper, 49, 51; horehound, 84; lemon balm, 90; meadow-sweet, 94; parsley, 99; pipsissewa, 101; thyme, 108.

flatulence — see angelica, 32; anise, 33; ginger, 72; peppermint, 97; valerian, 110; white mustard, 111.

flu (influenza) — see boneset, 46, goldenseal, 75.

insomnia — see chamomile, 52; dandelion, 61; lemon balm, 90; passion flower, 100; valerian, 109.

jaundice — see dandelion, 60; marigold, 92.

lice — see American hellebore, 31.

malaria — see echinacea, 62.

measles — see American hellebore, 31; echinacea, 62.

meningitis — see garlic, 67, 69.

menstrual cramps — see peppermint, 97.

motion sickness — see cayenne pepper, 49, 51; ginger, 72, 73.

multiple sclerosis — see cod-liver oil, 58.

nausea — see ginger, 72.

neuralgia — see parsley, 99; passion flower, 100.

obesity — see bladder wrack, 44, 45; kelp, 86.

pneumonia — see white mustard, 112.

psoriasis — see birch, 40; cod-liver oil, 57; gotu kola, 77.

rheumatism — see angelica, 32; arnica, 35; bay, 38; birch, 39, 40; boneset, 46; cod-liver oil, 57; dandelion, 61; feverfew, 66, 67; hops, 81-83; horehound, 84; juniper, 84; peppermint,

16

Kitchen-Cabinet Cures

from Grandma Bell's Journal

16 "Kitchen-Cabinet" Cures

from Grandma Bell's Journals

For too long, doctors in this country have given up their common sense — the very thing which I believe made this country what it is, or sadly, what it was — for the comfort of scientific theory. No thinking, just follow the company line. If patients suffer ... well, that's the price you pay for medical "progress." For years, I watched my colleagues ignore common sense evidence and make the most absurd diagnoses simply because they were more inclined to worship scientific procedures than to follow age-old wisdom.

Unfortunately, I did the same, until the weight of evidence and the weight on my heart forced me to look, for the first time, at the wisdom of traditional home remedies and the value of my own good old American common sense.

What a revelation! Once you wake up from the nightmare of scientific theology and clear your head of the constant propaganda spewing forth from greedy drug companies, reality hits hard and fast. My life (my medical life, I should say) took a turn for the better. In a way, I came home again — back to my early American pioneer roots and the wisdom of my grandmother, affectionately known to the Douglass clan as Grandma Bell.

That's what this pamphlet is all about — coming home. What I once believed to be old wives' tales — stories long destroyed by the new world of science — actually proved to be the best treatment for many of the common ailments you and I suffer through. So I put a few of them together in this booklet with the sincere hope that Grandma Bell's wisdom will help you recover your common sense, and take responsibility for your own health, the same way it did for me.

Now I'm not saying all of these natural remedies are viable in all cases. No one in his right mind would claim that. And you've certainly heard me say many times that certain illnesses require specific drugs — natural remedies won't do if you have pneumonia.

But it's not often, if at all, that natural remedies can cause harm. At their best, they solve your problem without dangerous drugs and drug-induced side effects. At worst, they don't work, but they don't usually harm you.

Oftentimes, this non-invasive, non-drug method is the first way to go. Before you spend $50 at your doctor's office and start taking expensive drugs, try the simplest method first. The human body is a wonder. It can repair itself, and usually does without intervention. In fact, many of the results we attribute to drugs are simply the body repairing itself. The drugs have little or nothing to do with it.

So, many times, the simplest way is the best. That's what I'm offering here — simple, common sense, tried and true remedies for that *oh so painful* ailment, that just *may* work for you.

Angina:

I'm convinced that angina has been around as long as man himself. You can read accounts of "sudden attacks of chest pain" in the writings of various Roman historians and philosophers. And like those who today suffer from angina, the experience is frightening.

Contemporary medicine seems to think it knows how to stop angina pain. Of course, the answer is drugs — powerful drugs with massive side effects.

Grandma Bell knew that angina is mostly triggered by smoking, eating, exertion, and anxiety. And with a bit of rest the pain dissipates. The cause of the pain is a lack of oxygen to the heart. Usually this lack of oxygen is caused by a hardening of the arteries.

In Grandma's days they knew that light exercise — walking, to be specific — could help reduce the frequency of angina attacks. What they also knew, perhaps instinctively, was that light exercise was and is a great way to reduce stress. Reduce stress, and you have a good chance of reducing angina.

One thing Grandma didn't know: If you suffer from angina and you are a smoker — you're on the road to a quick exit. If you stop smoking, you'll cut your chance of heart attack by 50%. Think about it!

Arthritis:

Let me say it up front — there is no known cure for rheumatoid arthritis. Grandma knew this 100 years ago, but we seem to have forgotten this fact in our rush to embrace contemporary medicine.

We simply can't admit defeat, so we keep trying magic pill after magic pill. Nothing works. Tell your doctor to quit wasting your time and money on useless, dangerous pills like Feldene.

When Grandma had arthritis she took an aspirin to reduce swelling. "Grandpa Bill" says do the same. Aspirin is cheaper than the arthritis drugs doctors are pushing today, and although aspirin is not without side effects, it beats the heck out of any other pill you can try.

Grandma knew nothing about steroids and you should follow her lead. Forget steroids — unless you want to end up with osteoporosis.

One thing the old girl knew: To reduce the pain of arthritis, *lose some weight*. Less weight means less stress on your bones.

Can diet affect the severity of arthritis? Definitely! If her arthritis got too bad, my grandmother would fast for a day or two. Funny, she never had any pain while fasting. She was quick enough to surmise that some of the foods she ate were helping to fuel the pain of arthritis. She was right.

Many arthritis suffers have complained to their doctors that certain foods definitely contributed to their symptoms. But mention arthritis and nutrition in one breath and you'll be labeled a quack in a heartbeat.

But the link is there. And a few brave researchers have shown that certain foods trigger a worsening of arthritis symptoms. Unfortunately, and as expected, there is no one trigger food. It's up to you to eliminate foods until you find which ones make your symptoms worse.

Start by eliminating wheat and rice products. If you feel better, add them again to your diet. If you feel worse, you've just performed a valuable scientific study which has yielded some accurate results. No reaction? Then try dairy products. With a bit of determination you'll be able to find the foods which spark your arthritis pain.

A recent study found that the omega-3 fatty acids found in fish oils had a positive effect in reducing tenderness of the joint. It's postulated that the omega-3 fatty acid, called EPA or eicosapentaenoic acid, helps reduce inflammation by stimulating the production of prostaglandins. Along with fish oil, "Grandpa Bill" also recommends taking between 500 - 1000 mg of vitamin C. *Note'*, I don't recommend more than 1000 mg of C a day.

I also recommend mild exercise. This is essential for reducing pain and slowing the deterioration of the joints. Hot baths help, and so does a gentle massage using an herbal potion which contains lemon.

Like most diseases, arthritis is worsened by the intake of white sugar. This stuff is poison — avoid it at all costs!

Finally, avoid iron supplements and multivitamins which contain iron. Among other things, excess iron can cause pain and swelling.

And if you're looking for an *avant garde,* yet effective natural treatment, try magnetic medicine. A recent Polish study found that joint pain and swelling were greatly reduced when an electrode is placed on the effected joint and a 25-minute electric pulse is given. There are no side effects, and the doctors report a 73-percent success rate with rheumatoid arthritis patients.

Constipation:

Constipation can be a serious business. In my opinion, some people worry about it too much; but for others it can be a painful problem.

There is some confusion, even among doctors, about exactly what constipation is. The elderly usually define it as a situation that requires straining to have a bowel movement, whereas doctors define it in terms of frequency. (As usual, the old folks are right.)

Just for the record: If you have a large movement, you don't need one every day, so don't worry one bit. A lot of people have only a few evacuations per week, and it never occurs to them that they might be constipated -they just have less reading time than the rest of us!

However, if you're absolutely sure you're corked-up, try one of these:

1. Don't do anything if you have gone only a few days without a movement. Things usually work out.

2. If waiting doesn't work, or it's too painful, drink four ounces of olive oil straight (if you're tough), or mixed in grapefruit juice.

3. A magnesium supplement, 500mgs a day, will often loosen things up. You should be taking at least this much magnesium for your health anyway.

4. One gram (1,000mg) of vitamin C will get things moving, too. The amount required may vary, especially if you're already C-deficient.

Coughs:

Do you want to depress your cough? If it's a useful or productive cough — meaning it is bringing up mucus — then the cough mechanism helps you expectorate all the gook in your bronchial tubes. If it collects there, you may get pneumonia. Prolonged suppression of the cough reflex can lead to bronchiectasis — pus pockets in the lungs. It's OK to take a little something at bed time to suppress the cough enough so that you can get some rest, but discontinue its use as soon as the cough abates. Hot lemon tea with honey is usually effective. See the section under sore throat for the Douglass Hot Toddy recipe which helps the cough and leaves you feeling no pain.

If it's a useless cough, then by all means take something to make it stop. Grandma had a theory about these useless kinds of coughs. She would always eat something salty. For some reason that seemed to stop the hacking cough. Another remedy was some licorice tea.

Many smokers come to me complaining that they had the flu but the cough won't go away. For what it's worth, I say, "Quit smoking." It's never well-received.

Diarrhea:

"Don't drink the water!" But if you've made the mistake of drinking what passes for water in parts of Spain, Mexico, Africa, and the Middle East, you know that diarrhea is one of the worst maladies you'll ever suffer through.

Grandma Bell had her own remedy — and it didn't involve antacids or Pepto Bismol. If the condition wasn't too severe, she would let it run its course, believing it was best to let the body eliminate the problem itself.

Grandma also believed in the calming power of chamomile tea. I heartily agree with her. And she always recommended eating, what she called, something "clear." Usually that meant chicken soup.

If the condition is too debilitating, I give my patients charcoal tablets (as many as four per hour until the diarrhea subsides). Charcoal helps absorb the bacteria and toxins that are causing the problem. And I recommend that my patients take high potency garlic capsules. Garlic is renown for its ability to kill bacteria and parasites.

Plus I suggest a good magnesium supplement (about 1000 mg per day) to help restore the body's proper pH balance.

Bottom line: If possible, let diarrhea run its course.

Earaches:

I don't know where Grandma got her information, but I certainly won't question it. She was convinced that mild earaches could be helped by going on a dairy free diet for a few days. Perhaps she thought the high protein content contributed to the problem. Whenever I had those typical kid's ears problems she would restrict my intake of dairy products and put a hot compress on my ear. In the evening, when she wanted me to sleep, she would use the compress and put a woollen hat over my head to keep the hot towel in place for the evening.

Grandma would always warn me not to blow my nose too violently. She was right, of course. Nose blowing, if it is done too violently, can help send the infection deeper into the ear.

Dr. Bill must warn that if there are symptoms of dizziness, ringing in the ears, loss of hearing, or a bloody discharge, it's time to see your doctor because there's a chance that the eardrum has ruptured.

Note: If ear wax is a problem, try a few drops of hydrogen peroxide. It will bubble in your ear and remove and soften the wax. It's cheaper than the over-the-counter remedies.

Fever:

Grandma Bell and Doctor Bill say leave the fever alone if it's under 102°F in adults and 103 °F in children. Fever is the body's way of fighting infection. Fever is not a disease, it's a symptom, and it helps the body fight what's ailing it.

With a cold or flu, the best remedy is sleep; consequently, if the fever and pain are keeping you from sleeping, take an aspirin at bedtime to help you sleep through the night. But do this only at bedtime; during the day let the fever take its course.

Never, never give aspirin to children!

Several herbal teas can help ease a fever. Grandma was big on licorice root and willow bark. We know today that willow bark contains lots of salicylates, which are related in chemical structure to aspirin.

Whenever I had a fever, Grandma always pushed juice on me. Now I'm pushing it on you. Natural fruit and vegetable juices are a good way to add needed liquid to your body and replace needed vitamins and minerals.

And finally, I heartily recommend taking a few garlic capsules. (Grandma used the cloves themselves — not a pretty picture.) Garlic, among many other things, is one of the world's first antibiotics and it helps power the immune system.

Fibrocystic Breast Disease:

Many women suffer from breast pain and tenderness each month. For some, each month brings the fear of breast cancer because suddenly a lump will appear, or maybe several lumps. One report even went so far as to say that 80 percent of women suffer from this condition at some time during their lives.

Many doctors don't believe it is a disease at all. It's a "normal condition for women of childbearing years." That's little comfort for those who are suffering.

And of course, if you go to your doctor complaining of lumps and pain, you'll be sent immediately for a mammogram —which I believe is a dangerous and expensive procedure.

If you find the pain and lumps to be cyclical — linked to your menstrual cycle — there's probably nothing to fear. And there are a few things you can do to help lessen the symptoms.

Research has shown that reducing your intake of caffeine — from tea, coffee, and chocolate —

can help control the condition. In one study, this approach worked in 66 percent of the women studied. It may work for you; it may not. But it does no harm to try. How many medical treatments can make that claim? Grandma Bill suggests that you give it a try and see if it works for you. Stop all caffeine-containing drugs and food for two to three months. If you notice a difference, you know you're on the right track.

Another option is to take vitamin E, 600 units a day for eight weeks. This approach works well for many women and has been used by enlightened physicians for many years. Again, it may work for you or it may not. But certainly there is no risk.

Finally, evening primrose oil has been found to be very effective in reducing the size of the lumps. I recommend two to three capsules daily.

It's important that women suffering from this problem religiously take a vitamin supplement which is high in vitamins E, A, and B-complex. One key is to take at least 10,000 units of beta-carotene daily.

Gum disease:

I read somewhere in the popular press that 90 percent of Americans suffer from some type of gum disease. Balderdash! It's a way to bring in millions of patients, and charge them upwards of

$5,000 each so that the gum doctors can vacation in Aruba and finance their winter homes in Palm Beach.

Most gum surgery is a ripoff — there, I've said it. Grandma's generation had no gum problems. I attribute this to the fact that there were few gum doctors in those days — and Grandma's contemporaries didn't brush their teeth with chemical goop.

Grandma knew that gum problems, if they did arise, could be easily treated with hydrogen peroxide. This therapy has been around since the 1700s.

The treatment consists of rubbing a mixture of baking soda and hydrogen peroxide into the gums. To make the treatment more effective you should first let your dentist do a basic cleanup around your teeth and gums, and you have to take the time to follow the procedure religiously.

Here's a typical story. Delores Dinapoli was diagnosed as having gum disease. She "went to a butcher[55] who cut up one fourth of her mouth. Another periodontist recommended still more surgery. She refused. Instead she turned to hydrogen peroxide. "After treatment my gums don't bleed or taste of pus; I have no pain or swelling."

Dr. Paul Cummings taught gum surgery at the University of North Carolina. Now he's converted to hydrogen peroxide therapy and reports a 98-percent success rate in 1,000 patients using the therapy.

"The irony is that you can get better results without surgery," says Cummings. "I've been using the non-surgical technique for five years and the results are 300 percent better than I ever got with surgery."

Grandma Bell could have told him that 50 years ago.

Heartburn/hiatal hernia:

Another plague of man. The older you get, the more your once favorite foods start to bother you. Maybe it's God's way of saying, "It's time you paid more attention to what you are eating."

Grandma suffered occasionally, as I do now, and she had a few rules when that burning sensation hit. First, she avoided coffee and tea; next, she quit taking the occasional nip (Grandma enjoyed a drink once in a while — "purely for medicinal purposes," she would say).

Your heartburn may not be caused by a hiatal hernia. Strange as it may sound, the heartburn could be caused by a lack of HCL — hydrochloric acid. Wait a minute, I can hear you say, how can that burning feeling be caused by a *lack* of stomach acid? HCL is needed to breakdown and digest a wide range of foods. If there's not enough

HCL the breakdown is incomplete, and heartburn can result.

Here's a test you can take. When heartburn strikes, take one teaspoon of apple cider vinegar or lemon juice. If the heartburn goes away, it's time for you to start taking an HCL supplement because you need more stomach acid. If the symptoms get worse, forget HCL.

For excess stomach acid, belching, etc. there's nothing better than a few charcoal tablets to help absorb the acid. I don't recommend charcoal as a steady supplement, but for those times when heartburn is driving you crazy, charcoal can give you fast relief.

Grandma always had two suggestions whenever heartburn was a continuing problem: (1) sleep with your head elevated (She was right because if your problem is a hiatal hernia, sleeping with the head raised will keep stomach acid from moving up and into the esophagus); (2) eat smaller meals more often (this makes complete digestion much easier).

I'll remind you to avoid carbonated drinks and coffee.

Hemorrhoids:

Not a laughing matter — unless you remember when Jimmy Carter couldn't function as president (when could he function?) because of his hemorrhoid surgery.

Bran works well to prevent flare-ups, but it can make things worse once an attack occurs. During an attack drink lots of water. After the attack try adding insoluble fiber to your diet. It takes a bit of experimentation to find the proper level of fiber intake. Not enough and there's no effect; too much and diarrhea sets in. So experiment until you find the amount that's right for you.

If you want to try one of Grandma's oldest remedies, peel -31 clove o{ yirUc, stripe k into ^ suppository 2ind vise it three times a week.

And remember, drink lots of pure water — not the chemical soup that flows from your tap!

Finally, don't forget to use your common sense: softer toilet tissue can help prevent some pain; don't go around lifting the refrigerator; take a hot bath to ease pain; don't scratch; and avoid spicy foods.

Osteoporosis:

Grandma's generation didn't know much about osteoporosis — it wasn't the "disease of the day" as it is now. Then again, in Grandma's day they didn't drink 50 gallons of carbonated beverages as the average American woman does today. And research has shown that there is a solid connection between carbonated beverage consumption and bone fractures in women.

One thing's for certain—calcium supplementation is not the way to go for the vast majority of women. It's becoming increasingly obvious that excess calcium intake may *cause* osteoporosis, not prevent it.

If you are concerned about osteoporosis the first thing to do is have a wholistic physician check you for a magnesium and manganese deficiency. Laboratory animals placed on a manganese-deficient diet had twice the osteoporosis as animals receiving a proper amount of the mineral. Manganese is hard for the body to absorb, so even foods that are rich in manganese may not be providing all that you need.

Shingles:

Grandma would recommend dabbing the blisters with hydrogen peroxide. I agree with her technique. Another technique I've used successfully is folic acid. I had a patient recently who suffered from severe, painful shingles near the belt line. The pain was so severe he could hardly stand. I put him on 25 mg of folic acid twice daily. When I saw him a week later, the pain was completely gone.

Sore throats:

Grandma's favorite recipe was slippery elm tea. There's nothing better to ease the pain. Slippery elm can be easily purchased at your local health food store.

Many of Grandma's friends swore by ginger tea. It's worth a try — especially if you don't like the taste of slippery elm.

If you want to try one of Grandma's real old remedies, you can try a chamomile poultice, wrapped around your throat with a warm cloth.

My recommendation is a bit more fun and less embarrassing. I happen to enjoy a Dr. Douglass Hot Toddy when my throat is on the fritz — a dash of lemon, some honey, and a good shot of whiskey. It works for me. After one or two the pain seems to subside.

During the past five years, there has been a growing body of research that validates the effectiveness of zinc gluconate lozenges in relieving sore throat and easing the general symptoms of a cold. The lozenges are now readily available. Take one every two hours until the sore throat subsides. Don't take the lozenges for more than one week at a time.

Ulcers:

Under the heading of Heartburn/Hiatal Hernia, I suggested a simple test to determine if your stomach has an excess or a deficiency of hydrochloric acid (HCL). If you believe you have an ulcer, I recommend that you perform this simple test with apple cider vinegar or lemon juice. If you have an excess of stomach acid consider drinking 4 oz. of aloe vera gel each day.

If you are deficient in HCL, do what Grandma did — sip apple cider vinegar and water with your meals.

If you have an ulcer, take my advice and avoid iron supplements. Iron is hard to digest and can cause a severe upset stomach in susceptible individuals.

Warts:

Grandma Bell's exhaustive list of treatments wouldn't be complete without a remedy or two for warts.

Here are a few of the most unique:
1. Crushed garlic placed directly on the wart and covered with a bandage for 24 hours.
2. Castor oil directly on the wart.
3. It's been argued that warts are caused by an excess of fat and protein being excreted. Sounds strange to me, but then again so do a lot of things.
4. Crush vitamin C tablets and put the paste on the wart. Why not?
5. Rub the wart with a raw potato.
6. Vitamin E oil placed on the pad of a bandage and wrapped around the wart. Replace the bandage daily until the wart is gone — usually about two weeks.

But here's my favorite: watermelon seeds. If you have warts eat a lot of watermelon and swallow the seeds. It works wonderfully well against warts.

Dr. Haines Ely from the University of California at Davis discovered this remarkable therapeutic use for the watermelon seed. At first he thought it was just the placebo effect — that influence of doctor over patient that makes the patient get well almost magically. But when his patients started treating their friends and neighbors with seeds, Dr. Ely knew the seeds were working on some pharmacologic level.

He hypothesizes that watermelon seeds, being a mild diuretic, flush out some compound that the wart needs to grow. A wart virus will not grow in a tissue culture, which indicates that some property is missing from the culture that is found in the human host.

So, give watermelon seeds a try. And if they work, please let me know.

Anyway, Grandma Bell would have been very proud of old Dr. Ely.

About Doctor William Campbell Douglass II

Dr. Douglass reveals medical truths, and deceptions, often at risk of being labeled heretical. He is consumed by a passion for living a long healthy life, and wants his readers to share that passion. Their health and well-being comes first. He is anti-dogmatic, and unwavering in his dedication to improve the quality of life of his readers. He has been called "the conscience of modern medicine," a "medical maverick," and has been voted "Doctor of the Year" by the National Health Federation. His medical experiences are far reaching-from battling malaria in Central America - to fighting deadly epidemics at his own health clinic in Africa - to flying with U.S. Navy crews as a flight surgeon - to working for 10 years in emergency medicine here in the States. These learning experiences, not to mention his keen storytelling ability and wit, make Dr. Douglass' newsletters (Daily Dose and Real Health) and books uniquely interesting and fun to read. He shares his no-frills, no-bull approach to health care, often amazing his readers by telling them to ignore many widely-hyped good-health practices (like staying away from red meat, avoiding coffee, and eating like a bird), and start living again by eating REAL food, taking some inexpensive supplements, and doing the pleasurable things that make life livable. Readers get all this, plus they learn how to burn fat, prevent cancer, boost libido, and so much more. And, Dr. Douglass is not afraid to challenge the latest studies that come out, and share the real story with his readers. Dr. William C. Douglass has led a colorful, rebellious, and crusading life. Not many physicians would dare put their professional reputations on the line as many times as this courageous healer has. A vocal opponent of "business-as-usual" medicine, Dr. Douglass has championed patients' rights and physician commitment to wellness throughout his career. This dedicated physician has repeatedly gone far beyond the call of duty in his work to spread the truth about alternative therapies. For a full year, he endured economic and physical hardship to work with physicians at the Pasteur Institute in St. Petersburg, Russia, where advanced research on photoluminescence was being conducted. Dr. Douglass comes from a distinguished family of physicians. He is the fourth generation Douglass to practice medicine, and his son is also a physician. Dr. Douglass graduated from the University of Rochester, the Miami School of Medicine, and the Naval School of Aviation and Space Medicine.

You want to protect those you love from the health dangers the authorities aren't telling you about, and learn the incredible cures that they've scorned and ignored?
Subscribe to the free Daily Dose updates "...the straight scoop about health, medicine, and politics." by sending an e-mail to real_sub@agoramail.net with the word "subscribe" in the subject line.

Dr. William Campbell Douglass'
Real Health:

Had Enough?

Enough turkey burgers and sprouts?

Enough forcing gallons of water down your throat?

Enough exercising until you can barely breathe?

Before you give up everything just because "everyone" says it's healthy...

Learn the facts from Dr. William Campbell Douglass, medicine's most acclaimed myth-buster. In every issue of Dr. Douglass' Real Health newsletter, you'll learn shocking truths about "junk medicine" and how to stay healthy while eating eggs, meat and other foods you love.

With the tips you'll receive from Real Health, you'll see your doctor less, spend a lot less money and be happier and healthier while you're at it. The road to Real Health is actually easier, cheaper and more pleasant than you dared to dream.

*Subscribe to Real Health today by calling 1-800-981-7162 or visit the Real Health web site at www.realhealthnews.com.
Use promotional code : DRHBDZZZ*

If you knew of a procedure that could save thousands, maybe millions, of people dying from AIDS, cancer, and other dreaded killers....

Would you cover it up?

It's unthinkable that what could be the best solution ever to stopping the world's killer diseases is being ignored, scorned and rejected. But that is exactly what's happening right now.

The procedure is called "photoluminescence". It's a thoroughly tested, proven therapy that uses the healing power of the light to perform almost miraculous cures.

This remarkable treatment works its incredible cures by stimulating the body's own immune responses. That's why it cures so many ailments--and why it's been especially effective against AIDS! Yet, 50 years ago, it virtually disappeared from the halls of medicine.

Why has this incredible cure been ignored by the medical authorities of this country? You'll find the shocking answer here in the pages of this new edition of Into the Light. Now available with the blood irradiation Instrument Diagram and a complete set of instructions for building your own "Treatment Device". Also includes details on how to use this unique medical instrument.

Rhino Publishing S.A.
www.rhinopublish.com

Into the Light

Into the Light

Dr. Douglass' Complete Guide to Better Vision

A report about eyesight and what can be done to improve it naturally. But I've also included information about how the eye works, brief descriptions of various common eye conditions, traditional remedies to eye problems, and a few simple suggestions that may help you maintain your eyesight for years to come.
-William Campbell Douglass II, MD

The Hypertension Report.
Say Good Bye to High Blood Pressure.

An estimated 50 million Americans have high blood pressure. Often called the "silent killer" because it may not cause symptoms until the patient has suffered serious damage to the arterial system. Diet, exercise, potassium supplements chelation therapy and practically anything but drugs is the way to go and alternatives are discussed in this report.

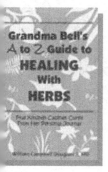

Grandma Bell's A To Z Guide To Healing With Herbs.

This book is all about - coming home. What I once believed to be old wives' tales - stories long destroyed by the new world of science - actually proved to be the best treatment for many of the common ailments you and I suffer through. So I put a few of them together in this book with the sincere hope that Grandma Bell's wisdom will help you recover your common sense, and take responsibility for your own health. -William Campbell Douglass II, MD

Prostate Problems:
Safe, Simple, Effective Relief for Men over 50.

Don't be frightened into surgery or drugs you may not need. First, get the facts about prostate problems... know all your options, so you can make the best decisions. This fully documented report explains the dangers of conventional treatments, and gives you alternatives that could save you more than just money!

Color me Healthy
The Healing Powers of Colors

"He's crazy!"
"He's got to be a quack!"
"Who gave this guy his medical license?"
"He's a nut case!"

In case you're wondering, those are the reactions you'll probably get if you show your doctor this report. I know the idea of healing many common ailments simply by exposing them to colored light sounds far-fetched, but when you see the evidence, you'll agree that color is truly an amazing medical breakthrough.

When I first heard the stories,
I reacted much the same way.
But the evidence so
convinced me, that I had to
try color therapy in my practice.
My results were truly amazing.

-William Campbell Douglass II, MD

Order your complete set of Roscolene filters (choice of 3 sizes) to be used with the "Color Me Healthy" therapy. The eleven Roscolene filters are # 809, 810, 818, 826, 828, 832, 859, 861, 866, 871, and 877. The filters come with protective separator sheets between each filter. The color names and the Roscolene filter(s) used to produce that particular color, are printed on a card included with the filters and a set of instructions on how to fit them to a lamp.

Rhino Publishing
www.rhinopublish.com

What Is Going on Here?

Peroxides are supposed to be bad for you. Free radicals and all that. But now we hear that hydrogen peroxide is good for us. Hydrogen peroxide will put extra oxygen in your blood. There's no doubt about that. Hydrogen peroxide costs pennies. So if you can get oxygen into the blood cheaply and safely, maybe cancer (which doesn't like oxygen), emphysema, AIDS, and many other terrible diseases can be treated effectively. Intravenous hydrogen peroxide rapidly relieves allergic reactions, influenza symptoms, and acute viral infections.

No one expects to live forever. But we would all like to have a George Burns finish. The prospect of finishing life in a nursing home after abandoning your tricycle in the mobile home park is not appealing. Then comes the loss of control of vital functions the ultimate humiliation. Is life supposed to be from tricycle to tricycle and diaper to diaper? You come into this world crying, but do you have to leave crying? I don't believe you do. And you won't either after you see the evidence. Sounds too good to be true, doesn't it? Read on and decide for yourself.

-William Campbell Douglass II, MD

Rhino Publishing S.A.
www.rhinopublish.com

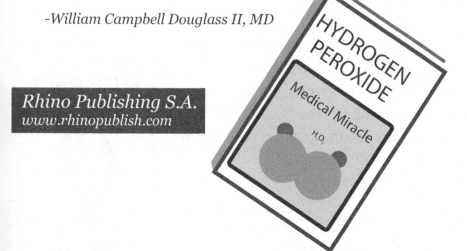

HYDROGEN PEROXIDE

Medical Miracle

H_2O

Don't drink your milk!

If you knew what we know about milk... BLEECHT! All that pasteurization, homogenization and processing is not only cooking all the nutrients right out of your favorite drink. It's also adding toxic levels of vitamin D.

This fascinating book tells the whole story about milk. How it once was nature's perfect food...how "raw," unprocessed milk can heal and boost your immune system ... why you can't buy it legally in this country anymore, and what we could do to change that.

Dr. "Douglass traveled all over the world, tasting all kinds of milk from all kinds of cows, poring over dusty research books in ancient libraries far from home, to write this light-hearted but scientifically sound book.

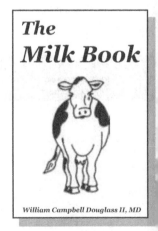

The
Milk Book

William Campbell Douglass II, MD

Rhino Publishing, S.A.
www.rhinopublish.com

Eat Your Cholesterol!

Eat Meat, Drink Milk, Spread The Butter- And Live Longer!
How to Live off the Fat of the Land and Feel Great.

Americans are being saturated with anti-cholesterol propaganda. If you watch very much television, you're probably one of the millions of Americans who now has a terminal case of cholesterol phobia. The propaganda is relentless and is often designed to produce fear and loathing of this worst of all food contaminants. You never hear the food propagandists bragging about their product being fluoride-free or aluminum-free, two of our truly serious food-additive problems. But cholesterol, an essential nutrient, not proven to be harmful in any quantity, is constantly pilloried as a menace to your health. If you don't use corn oil, Fleischmann's margarine, and Egg Beaters, you're going straight to atherosclerosis hell with stroke, heart attack, and premature aging -- and so are your kids. Never feel guilty about what you eat again! Dr. Douglass shows you why red meat, eggs, and dairy products aren't the dietary demons we're told they are. But beware: This scientifically sound report goes against all the "common wisdom" about the foods you should eat. Read with an open mind.

Rhino Publishing, S.A.
www.rhinopublish.com

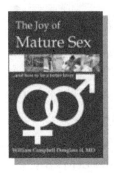

The Joy of Mature Sex and How to Be a Better Lover

Humans are very confused about what makes good sex. But I believe humans have more to offer each other than this total licentiousness common among animals. We're talking about mature sex. The kind of sex that made this country great.

Stop Aging or Slow the Process How Exercise With Oxygen Therapy (EWOT) Can Help

EWOT (pronounced ee-watt) stands for Exercise With Oxygen Therapy. This method of prolonging your life is so simple and you can do it at home at a minimal cost. When your cells don't get enough oxygen, they degenerate and die and so you degenerate and die. It's as simple as that.

Hormone Replacement Therapies: Astonishing Results For Men And Women

It is accurate to say that when the endocrine glands start to fail, you start to die. We are facing a sea change in longevity and health in the elderly. Now, with the proper supplemental hormones, we can slow the aging process and, in many cases, reverse some of the signs and symptoms of aging.

Add 10 Years to Your Life With some "best of" Dr. Douglass' writings.

To add ten years to your life, you need to have the right attitude about health and an understanding of the health industry and what it's feeding you. Following the established line on many health issues could make you very sick or worse! Achieve dynamic health with this collection of some of the "best of" Dr. Douglass' newsletters.

How did AIDS become one of the Greatest Biological Disasters in the History of Mankind?

GET THE FACTS

AIDS and BIOLOGICAL WARFARE covers the history of plagues from the past to today's global confrontation with AIDS, the Prince of Plagues. Completely documented *AIDS and BIOLOGICAL WARFARE* helps you make your own decisions about how to survive in a world ravaged by this horrible plague.

You will learn that AIDS is not a naturally occuring disease process as you have been led to believe, but a man-made biological nightmare that has been unleashed and is now threatening the very existence of human life on the planet.

There is a smokescreen of misinformation clouding the AIDS issue. Now, for the first time, learn the truth about the nature of the crisis our planet faces: its origin -- how AIDS is really transmited and alternatives for treatment. Find out what they are not telling you about AIDS and Biological Warfare, and how to protect yourself and your loved ones. AIDS is a serious problem worldwide, but it is no longer the major threat. You need to know the whole story. To protect yourself, you must know the truth about biological warfare.

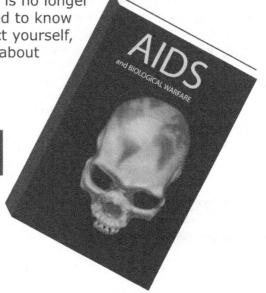

Rhino Publishing S.A.
www.rhinopublish.com

PAINFUL DILEMMA

Are we fighting the wrong war?

We are spending millions on the war against drugs while we
should be fighting the war against pain with those drugs!

As you will read in this book, the war on drugs was lost a long time ago and,
when it comes to the war against pain, pain is winning! An article in USA Today
(11/20/02) reveals that dying patients are not getting relief from pain. It seems
the doctors are torn between fear of the government, certainly justified, and a
clinging to old and out dated ideas about pain, which is NOT justified.

A group called Last Acts, a coalition of health-care groups, has released a very
discouraging study of all 50 states that nearly half of the 1.6 million Americans
living in nursing homes suffer from untreated pain. They said that life was being
extended but it amounted to little more than "extended pain and suffering."

This book offers insight into the history of pain treatment and the current failed
philosophies of contemporary medicine. Plus it describes some of today's most
advanced treatments for alleviating certain kinds of pain. This book is not another
"self-help" book touting home remedies; rather, Painful Dilemma: Patients in
Pain -- People in Prison, takes a hard look at where we've gone wrong and what
we (you) can do to help a loved one who is living with chronic pain.

The second half of this book is a must read if you value your freedom. We now
have the ridiculous and tragic situation of people
in pain living in a government-created hell by
restriction of narcotics and people in prison for
trying to bring pain relief by the selling of
narcotics to the suffering. The end result of the
"war on drugs" has been to create the greatest
and most destructive cartel in history, so great,
in fact, that the drug Mafia now controls most
of the world economy.

Rhino Publishing S.A.
www.rhinopublish.com

Live the Adventure!

Why would anyone in their right mind put everything they own in storage and move to Russia, of all places?! But when maverick physician Bill Douglass left a profitable medical practice in a peaceful mountaintop town to pursue "pure medical truth".... none of us who know him well was really surprised.

After All, anyone who's braved the outermost reaches of darkest Africa, the mean streets of Johannesburg and New York, and even a trip to Washington to testify before the Senate, wouldn't bat and eye at ducking behind the Iron Curtain for a little medical reconnaissance!

Enjoy this imaginative, funny, dedicated man's tales of wonder and woe as he treks through a year in St. Petersburg, working on a cure for the world's killer diseases. We promise --

YOU WON'T BE BORED!

Rhino Publishing S.A.
www.rhinopublish.com

THE SMOKER'S PARADOX
THE HEALTH BENEFITS OF TOBACCO!

The benefits of smoking tobacco have been common knowledge for centuries. From sharpening mental acuity to maintaining optimal weight, the relatively small risks of smoking have always been outweighed by the substantial improvement to mental and physical health. Hysterical attacks on tobacco notwithstanding, smokers always weigh the good against the bad and puff away or quit according to their personal preferences. Now the same anti-tobacco enterprise that has spent billions demonizing the pleasure of smoking is providing additional reasons to smoke. Alzheimer's, Parkinson's, Tourette's Syndrome, even schizophrenia and cocaine addiction are disorders that are alleviated by tobacco. Add in the still inconclusive indication that tobacco helps to prevent colon and prostate cancer and the endorsement for smoking tobacco by the medical establishment is good news for smokers and non-smokers alike. Of course the revelation that tobacco is good for you is ruined by the pharmaceutical industry's plan to substitute the natural and relatively inexpensive tobacco plant with their overpriced and ineffective nicotine substitutions. Still, when all is said and done, the positive revelations regarding tobacco are very good reasons indeed to keep lighting those cigars - but only 4 a day!

Rhino Publishing, S.A
www.rhinopublish.com

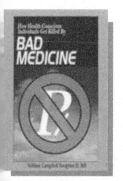

Bad Medicine
How Individuals Get Killed By Bad Medicine.

Do you really need that new prescription or that overnight stay in the hospital? In this report, Dr. Douglass reveals the common medical practices and misconceptions endangering your health. Best of all, he tells you the pointed (but very revealing!) questions your doctor prays you never ask. Interesting medical facts about popular remedies are revealed.

Dangerous Legal Drugs
The Poisons in Your Medicine Chest.

If you knew what we know about the most popular prescription and over-the-counter drugs, you'd be sick. That's why Dr. Douglass wrote this shocking report about the poisons in your medicine chest. He gives you the low-down on different categories of drugs. Everything from painkillers and cold remedies to tranquilizers and powerful cancer drugs.

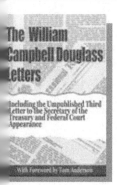

The William Campbell Douglass Letters.
Expose of Government Machinations
(Vietnam War).

THE WILLIAM CAMPBELL DOUGLASS LETTERS. Dr. Douglass' Defense in 1968 Tax Case and Expose of Government Machinations during the Vietnam War.

The Eagle's Feather. A Novel of
International Political Intrigue.

Although The Eagle's Feather is a work of fiction set in the 1970's, it is built, as with most fiction, on a framework of plausibility and background information. This is a fiction book that could not have been written were it not for various ominous aspects, which pose a clear and present danger to the security of the United States.

Rhino Publishing

ORDER FORM

PURCHASER INFORMATION

Purchaser's Name (Please Print): _____

Shipping Address (Do not use a P.O. Box): _____

City: _____ State/Prov.: _____ Country: _____

Zip/Postal Code: _____ Telephone No.: _____ Fax No.: _____

E-Mail Address (if interested in receiving free e-Books when available): _____

CREDIT CARD INFO (CIRCLE ONE):

MASTERCARD, VISA, AMERICAN EXPRESS, DISCOVER, JCB, DINER'S CLUB, CARTE BLANCHE.

Charge my Card -> Number #: _____ Exp.: _____

*Security Code: _____ * Required for all MasterCard, Visa and American Express purchases. For your security, we require that you enter your card's verification number. The verification number is also called a CCV number. This code is the 3 digits farthest right on the back of your VISA/MC, or the 4 digits to the right on the front of your American Express card. Your credit card statement will show **a different name than Rhino Publishing** as the vendor.

WE DO NOT share your private information, we use 3ʳᵈ party credit card processing service to process your order only.

ADDITIONAL INFORMATION

If your shipping address is not the same as your credit card billing address, please indicate your card billing address here.

_____   _____
Name on the card   Type of card:

Billing Address: _____

City: _____   State/Prov.: _____   Zip/Postal Code: _____

Fax a copy of this order to:
RHINO PUBLISHING, S.A.
1-888-317-6767 or International #: + 416-352-5126

To order by mail, send your payment by first class mail only to the following address. Please include a copy of this order form. Make your check or bank drafts (NO postal money order) payable to RHINO PUBLISHING, S.A. and mail to:

Rhino Publishing, S.A.
Attention: PTY 5048
P.O. Box 025724
Miami, FL.
USA 33102

Digital E-books also available online: www.rhinopublish.com

Rhino Publishing

ORDER FORM

Purchaser's Name (Please Print): _____

I would like to order the following paperback book of Dr. Douglass (Alternative Medicine Books):

___	X	9962-636-04-3	Add 10 Years to Your Life. With some "best of" Dr. Douglass writings.	$13.99 $____
___	X	9962-636-07-8	AIDS and Biological Warfare. What They Are Not Telling You!	$17.99 $____
___	X	9962-636-09-4	Bad Medicine. How Individuals Get Killed By Bad Medicine.	$11.99 $____
___	X	9962-636-10-8	Color Me Healthy. The Healing Power of Colors.	$11.99 $____
___	X	9962-636-XX-X	Color Filters for Color Me Healthy. 11 Basic Roscolene Filters for Lamps.	$21.89 $____
___	X	9962-636-15-9	Dangerous Legal Drugs. The Poisons in Your Medicine Chest.	$13.99 $____
___	X	9962-636-18-3	Dr. Douglass' Complete Guide to Better Vision. Improve eyesight naturally.	$11.99 $____
___	X	9962-636-19-1	Eat Your Cholesterol! How to Live off the Fat of the Land and Feel Great.	$11.99 $____
___	X	9962-636-12-4	Grandma Bell's A To Z Guide To Healing. Her Kitchen Cabinet Cures.	$14.99 $____
___	X	9962-636-22-1	Hormone Replacement Therapies. Astonishing Results For Men & Women	$11.99 $____
___	X	9962-636-25-6	Hydrogen Peroxide: One of the Most Underused Medical Miracle.	$15.99 $____
___	X	9962-636-27-2	Into the Light. New Edition with Blood Irradiation Instrument Instructions.	$19.99 $____
___	X	9962-636-54-X	Milk Book. The Classic on the Nutrition of Milk and How to Benefit from it.	$17.99 $____

___	X	9962-636-00-0	Painful Dilemma - Patients in Pain - People in Prison.	$17.99	$ ___
___	X	9962-636-32-9	Prostate Problems. Safe, Simple, Effective Relief for Men over 50.	$11.99	$ ___
___	X	9962-636-34-5	St. Petersburg Nights. Enlightening Story of Life and Science in Russia.	$17.99	$ ___
___	X	9962-636-37-X	Stop Aging or Slow the Process. Exercise With Oxygen Therapy Can Help.	$11.99	$ ___
___	X	9962-636-60-4	The Hypertension Report. Say Good Bye to High Blood Pressure.	$11.99	$ ___
___	X	9962-636-48-5	The Joy of Mature Sex and How to Be a Better Lover...	$13.99	$ ___
___	X	9962-636-43-4	The Smoker's Paradox: Health Benefits of Tobacco.	$14.99	$ ___

Political Books:

___	X	9962-636-40-X	The Eagle's Feather. A 70's Novel of International Political Intrigue.	$15.99	$ ___
___	X	9962-636-46-9	The W. C. D. Letters. Expose of Government Machinations (Vietnam War).	$11.99	$ ___

SUB-TOTAL: $ ___

ADD $5.00 HANDLING FOR YOUR ORDER: $ 5.00 $ 5.00

___ X ADD $2.50 SHIPPING FOR EACH ITEM ON ORDER: $ 2.50 $ ___

NOTE THAT THE MINIMUM SHIPPING AND HANDLING IS $7.50 FOR 1 BOOK ($5.00 + $2.50)
For order shipped outside the US, add $5.00 per item

___ X ADD $5.00 S. & H. OR EACH ITEM ON ORDER (INTERNATIONAL ORDERS ONLY) $ 5.00 $ ___
Allow up to 21 days for delivery (we will call you about back orders if any)

TOTAL: $ ___

Fax a copy of this order to: 1-888-317-6767 or Int'l + 416-352-5126
or mail to: Rhino Publishing, S.A. Attention: PTY 5048 P.O. Box 025724, Miami, FL., 33102 USA
Digital E-books also available online: www.rhinopublish.com

Made in United States
Orlando, FL
22 November 2024

54306876R00095